Life's Little Emergencies

A Handbook for Active Independent Seniors and Caregivers

Rod Brouhard, BBA, EMT-P

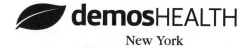
demosHEALTH

New York

Visit our website at www.demoshealth.com

ISBN: 978-1-936303-15-1
E-book ISBN: 9781617050749

Acquisitions Editor: Noreen Henson
Compositor: Absolute Service Inc.

Medical information provided by Demos Health, in the absence of a visit with a health care professional, must be considered as an educational service only. This book is not designed to replace a physician's independent judgment about the appropriateness or risks of a procedure of therapy for a given patient. Our purpose is to provide you with information that will help you make your own health care decisions.

The information and opinions provided here are believed to be accurate and sound, based on the best judgment available to the authors, editors, and publisher, but readers who fail to consult appropriate health authorities assume the risk of injuries. The publisher is not responsible for errors or omissions. The editors and publisher welcome any reader to report to the publisher any discrepancies or inaccuracies noticed.

Library of Congress Cataloging-in-Publication Data
CIP data is available from the Library of Congress.

Special discounts on bulk quantities of Demos Health books are available to corporations, professional associations, pharmaceutical companies, health care organizations, and other qualifying groups. For details, please contact:

Special Sales Department
Demos Medical Publishing
11 West 42nd Street, 15th Floor
New York, NY 10036
Phone: 800-532-8663 or 212-683-0072
Fax: 212-941-7842
E-mail: rsantana@demosmedpub.com

Printed in the United States of America by Bang Printing.
11 12 13 14 / 5 4 3 2 1

Contents

SECTION II.   SAVING LIVES

SECTION III.   INJURIES AND ILLNESSES

Foreword

Everyone needs a "go-to" person in their daily lives. Though many of us are lucky to have one, not everyone has such access. Now everyone can turn to Rod Brouhard, an experienced and perceptive emergency medical technician, a *go-to guy* with the skill to distill complex concepts into language that everyone can absorb.

Life's Little Emergencies is an informative, easy-to-understand guide that is both a first aid manual and a trusted go-to friend. The information contained in *Life's Little Emergencies* guides someone in simple tasks, such as how to evaluate and dress a wound effectively. It is very clear when *not* to use the guide in place of a trained and well-equipped first responder. It explains what you should do as well as what to expect after a trained first responder arrives.

This book is clear, concise, and a bit irreverent. It is fun to read. Its format supports remembering the important points for more than a short time.

Although the book is directed at seniors, it really has a much wider audience. For the few remaining schools that teach *health* or for a business that is not large enough to have an employee health service, *Life's Little Emergencies* should be mandatory reading and subject to regular review like fire or evacuation drills.

Stewart B. Fleishman MD,
author of *Learn to Live Through Cancer: What You Need to Know and Do* and the *Manual of Cancer Treatment Recovery: What the Practitioner Needs to Know and Do*

I
Getting Started

1

Is This an Emergency?

Who Should I Call?

Passed Out?
Weak on One Side?
Won't Wake Up?
Squirting Blood?
Short of Breath?
No Longer Moving?

YES → **CALL 911**

NO → **Keep Reading**

J ust in case you pulled this book off the shelf to help you in an emergency, here are six reasons to put it down right now and call 911:

- *Passing out.* If someone has suddenly passed out (lost consciousness), call 911.
- *Weakness on one side.* If only one hand is working correctly or only half of your pearly whites show up when you try to smile, call 911 immediately. If it turns out to be a stroke, the clock is already ticking.
- *Won't wake up.* If someone won't wake up, even after giving him or her a vigorous rub on the sternum (breastbone) with your knuckles (hard enough to hurt), call 911.
- *Bright red blood that won't stop squirting.* If there's blood squirting from a wound and you can't make it stop, call 911.
- *Sudden shortness of breath.* If someone is having trouble breathing right now that he or she didn't have a few minutes ago (especially if that person complains of itching or develops a bumpy rash), call 911.
- *Someone isn't moving after getting hurt (punched, fell, struck by a car, etc.).* Don't move the person unless he or she needs cardiopulmonary resuscitation (CPR; Chapter 8).

Assuming these emergencies aren't happening right now, I encourage you to read on.

FOLLOW YOUR GUT

When I take the ambulance to visit kindergarten classes to talk to the kids, I will ask them if they know the number to call in an emergency. They always do. One hundred 6-year-olds screaming "nine-one-one" in unison is pretty deafening.

Of course, learning a three-digit emergency telephone number is the easy part. Knowing when to use it is much tougher.

Asking those same 6-year-olds to describe an emergency produces mixed results:

"When the house is on fire."

"If my mom is sleeping on the couch."

"When our dog is having puppies."

"When a bad guy is trying to kill you." (I wonder about the dreams or nightmares of some of these kids.)

"When I fall off my bike."

Adults have just as much trouble deciding when to call 911 as kids do. In fact, I think adults tend to overanalyze incidents, which makes it even harder for them to recognize emergencies. Using your gut is a good first rule for deciding when to call 911.

When we're young, we work on instinct. If doing something made us uncomfortable, we didn't do it—unless we were told to do it by an adult. As we grow older, we're encouraged to ignore our gut feelings and to do things that make us nervous. Public speaking is a good example. Despite being the most feared activity, people still speak publicly, even those who don't really want to. Why do we do it? Because we have to. We'd rather not, but we ignore our fear and do it anyway.

We learn as we get older that it's not polite to refuse certain things— like a hug from creepy Uncle Joe (apologies to all the non-creepy Uncle Joes). We don't want to, but we're expected to.

As we age, we begin to weigh one choice, like how uncomfortable Uncle Joe makes us feel, against the other, like how uncomfortable it is to refuse his hug. Instead of following our gut instincts, we rationalize our decisions to fit what is expected of us.

Emergencies, by definition, are not expected. We don't plan them, and we aren't sure what to do with them. Because we don't have a plan, we can't rationalize our way through them. Emergencies are the part of our lives we need to guide with instinct; we need to follow our gut.

ALL EMERGENCIES ARE NOT CREATED EQUAL

Serious medical emergencies happen in real time with dire consequences unless the right decisions are made quickly. Brain damage, for example, begins about 4 minutes after the heart stops beating. Starting chest compressions (pushing on the chest during CPR) within that 4-minute window may make the difference between survival and death. It may also make the difference between surviving as a vegetable and surviving as a functional human being.

The six examples at the beginning of this chapter aren't the only times 911 should or could be called. Rather, they are the examples of when 911 must be called *now*, without delay.

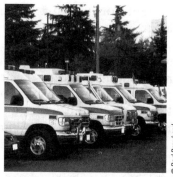

Most injuries or illnesses are not dire emergencies. They won't kill you if you don't act immediately. More often than not, the other stuff can wait a few minutes for us to get our wits about us—for us to analyze a little bit.

Each situation is different, and there are lots of reasons why folks call for an ambulance. Some of those reasons don't have much to do with how bad the emergency is. Every day in this country, ambulances deliver people to the hospital simply because they had no other means to get there. In the future there may be better ways to utilize emergency resources, but for now that's how the system works.

Should I NOT Call?

Not every injury or illness in need of first aid is also in need of emergency medical services. There are times when you don't need to call 911. There are also times when you don't even need to see a doctor.

In general, it's really hard to educate the public on when *not* to call 911. I would hate for you to agonize over a decision just to find out you should've summoned an ambulance. Remember, follow your gut. If you think you're in the midst of a medical emergency, call 911. If you aren't sure, but *think* you may be in the midst of a medical emergency, look it up—or just call 911.

It is the job of the ambulance and emergency department crews to determine if patients are truly experiencing serious illness or injuries. Basically, it's the job of the paramedics, emergency medical technicians (EMTs), doctors, and nurses to prioritize—we call it *triage*. Those with the most serious medical conditions will be treated first, little less serious next, and on down the line to the mildest conditions, which will be treated last.

Triage is the reason you can wait in the emergency department waiting room for hours when your medical condition warrants it. As more serious cases are brought to the emergency department for treatment, they are placed at the front of the line.

So, although I'll never discourage anyone from calling 911, it's only fair to warn you that minor medical conditions will be triaged by the responding ambulance crew and the emergency department staff. They'll evaluate your complaint and your physical signs to determine if you need immediate assistance or if you can wait.

If you aren't sure your condition is an emergency (or the condition of the person you are helping), then call 911, but be prepared to wait if your case is determined to be minor.

There are certainly situations needing first aid that may not need further medical treatment. With proper treatment, most abrasions (scrapes or scratches) won't need to be seen by a doctor unless they get infected. There are plenty of conditions that can wait for a private physician—even if it takes a day or two for an appointment.

Who You Gonna Call? (More Importantly, Who's Gonna Come?)

When I respond to calls for help in my day job as a paramedic, folks are often surprised by the number of rescuers that walk in the door. In my town, the fire department responds with the ambulance to most 911 calls. Five, and sometimes six, personnel arrive to every emergency call.

When you call 911 for a medical emergency, you may not only get an ambulance. Depending on where you live and how the emergency medical services (EMS) system is configured, you may also get the fire department or some sort of first-responder squad. Occasionally even the cops act as medical first responders, but that's very rare.

First responders are dispatched to an emergency to provide first aid in advance of the ambulance's arrival. Some first responders provide rescue operations (like cutting cars open to release pinned occupants). First responders also provide extra hands when necessary.

How to Use This Book

The first section of this book is about recognizing medical emergencies, getting the help you need, stocking the right kind of gear, and learning to work with first responders. *First aid* implies that the person with a medical emergency needs aid *now*, before more advanced medical care. Knowing how to get the help you need is just as important as what to do until help gets there.

We get down to saving lives in Section II. These are the most important procedures in the book. You can bet that if you need to do any of these things, you'll also be calling 911.

Section III contains a to-do list of injuries and conditions requiring first aid, and the procedures to treat them. Each condition, complaint, or procedure starts with a list of your priorities. You'll be told if seeking medical help is necessary, and instructed whether to call 911, your doctor, or do it yourself.

Section IV talks about surviving the environment we live in. This book is meant mostly for people to use on a day-to-day basis, but sometimes the environment comes to you whether you want it to or not.

This book is intended for you to use to take care of yourself or your family, which is why it jumps right into discussing the care given to loved ones. All of the advice, however, is perfectly good for your neighbors, students, teammates, classmates, inmates, or whomever you would like to help. Chapter 7 explains the legalities of helping others.

WHEN IN DOUBT, CALL 'EM OUT!

Listen to your gut.

Deciding if something is an emergency worthy of a call to 911 happens with each individual incident, and cannot be taught very easily. There are the six reasons listed at the beginning of this chapter:

- Passing out
- Weakness on one side
- Won't wake up
- Bright red blood that won't stop squirting
- Sudden shortness of breath
- Someone isn't moving after getting hurt

There are also all the procedures, conditions, and injuries listed in this book that include advice to call 911. For any situation, whether it's included in this book or not, always do more rather than less. If you're questioning whether to call 911 or not, then it is best to call.

When in doubt, call us out!

ON THE INTERNET

- firstaid.about.com/od/callingforhelp/qt/whentocall
- www.911.gov/whencall

2

The 411 About 911

- What will 911 ask me?
- How can I make sure they find me?
- Is it better to call 911 on a cell phone than on a landline?

If you're reading this book, you may no doubt remember back to the days when 911 didn't exist; while at the same time your grandkids (or great-grandkids) may have never seen a phone with a rotary dial. My wife and I have a rotary dial phone on our desk at home. When we first got it, the kids asked us how to dial the numbers; they thought maybe you were supposed to just push the holes like buttons. Once we showed them how it was done, one of them said, "That's why they call it *dialing*!"

The service 911 has been around since the late 1960s. It was a good idea: an easy-to-remember number to call in any emergency. The feds wanted to model it after the British 999 system. Ma Bell at the time already had 411 for information and 611 for line trouble, so 911 was born.

Calling 911 during an emergency sounds like a simple thing to do. You pick up the phone, push 9, then push 1 twice, and wait for someone to answer.

Then what? It's a stressful time. There are lives at stake and someone needs to be here pronto. Do you know what the 911 folks are going to say? Will you be prepared for what they're going to ask you?

WHAT TO EXPECT FROM 911

The 911 operators are known as *call takers*. They answer emergency lines and take down the information that emergency crews will need in order to find you in a hurry. In most parts of the country, 911 call takers are also certified to give you medical instructions before the flashing red lights show up in the driveway.

There are two questions that begin every 911 call:

- What is the location of the emergency?
- What phone number are you calling from?

There's a good reason for both of these. First of all, if you hang up, or the phone's battery goes dead, or a meteor falls from the heavens and destroys the phone lines 10 seconds into your 911 call, at least the call taker knows where to send help. He or she might not know what to send to you (ambulance, fire engine, or cop car) but you'll get somebody in a uniform with flashing lights on top of his or her vehicle and a radio that he or she can use to call in reinforcements.

Plus, if you get as far as giving your phone number before the line goes dead, the call taker at least has a number that he or she can try calling back.

In some parts of the country, the first question will be something like: "What is the nature of the emergency?" That's because the communication center that answers the phone might not be sending out all the troops. The communication center might need to transfer your call to another center depending on what type of help you need (medical, police, or fire). It's a good bet, however, that when the next call taker answers the line, the first question will be: "What is the location of the emergency?"

WHAT YOU MUST KNOW ABOUT CALLING 911

Whatever you do, stay on the line.

Expect the first two questions (which might be asked several times) to be: "Where are you?" and "What number are you calling from?"

Call from a landline (building phone) rather than a cell phone if you have the choice.

If you do call from a cell phone, tell them where you are and what kind of help you need right away.

Any cell phone that turns on and has a signal can call 911, but cell phones without contracts will not have a number for the 911 center to call you back if they need to.

Technology is an amazing thing and I'm sure right now you're thinking that 911 centers around the country have computers to tell them where you are. I mean, isn't that why you pay the extra 911 tax on your phone bill?

It's true. The ability of computers to tell the call taker your address is called E911 or enhanced 911. It's a pretty cool feature and it does work—most of the time. One of the reasons the call taker will ask your address and number, however, is because computers don't always get it right.

Tips to Get the Help You Need

Call takers and dispatchers only know what you tell them. They're taught to ask questions in a particular way, which may sound peculiar to you. If it doesn't make sense, tell them. They won't be offended.

The reason you called 911 was to get some help, and working with the call taker—rather than getting frustrated with him or her—is the best way to get that help. There are three things to remember whenever you call 911:

1. Don't hang up until the call taker tells you to. There are going to be lots of pauses when the call taker is talking to you. He or she is typing your answers into the computer, sending messages to other call takers and dispatchers, and might even be dispatching emergency crews over the radio. Indeed, it may seem like the call taker isn't on the line anymore, but chances are, he or she is. If you hang up too early, you might delay the emergency crews or miss some very important instructions.
2. Have patience with the call taker. This is your emergency. You need help and would be very happy if it showed up yesterday. You feel desperate and nobody seems to care. The call taker is going to do his or her best to walk you through the process and if you are impatient, the call taker is going to be stern with you to get the call under control. Remember, there's more than one person at the 911 center, so somebody is sending you help even though the call taker is still on the phone with you.
3. There are plenty of devices available that are designed to help you get help. I'm a believer that good old 911 is the best of the best, but that doesn't mean there aren't some good services on the market.

911 on the Go: Cell Phones

When I was a kid, the only phone we had was at the end of a wire coming out of the wall (and it had that dial on it). In fact, my mom had a phone in the laundry closet that had a giant coiled cord on the handset so she could talk to my aunt while doing the dishes or cooking dinner.

When cordless phones came out, we were ecstatic. It meant we no longer had to be attached to the kitchen or the office to talk to our friends. We could even go outside!

The only people with truly mobile phones—phones in their cars or in a briefcase—were rich corporate moguls or the president. (President Reagan's assistant would carry his cell phone in a saddlebag when the president went on horseback rides.)

Now, everybody's got a cellular phone. I'll bet your grandkids have cellular phones. I've seen kids in second grade with cell phones. I won't be surprised when they come out with dog cell phones (cats are too independent; they don't need them).

The problem with cell phones is when you need help. Cell phones aren't attached to the building, so that means they aren't attached to an address. When you call 911 from a phone in a building (we call that kind of phone a *landline*), if you don't know the address, the 911 call taker can figure it out. That doesn't really happen with a cell phone.

THE DIFFERENCE BETWEEN A CORDLESS PHONE AND A CELL PHONE

We live in a cordless world: remote controls, wireless Internet, and the little button that unlocks your car. With all the different phones out there, it might be tempting to refer to any phone without a cord as a cordless phone. But alas, a cordless phone is not the same as a cell phone or wireless phone.

Both do not have cords (or wires, for that matter). They can both be used to order a pizza, talk to the grandkids, or call an ambulance. The difference is in how they work.

Cordless phones work in a building. Although they're not cordless per se, they talk to a base that is plugged into a telephone jack on the wall. Imagine a cordless phone having an invisible string tying it to the house. It might work outside, but it won't go too far. If you call 911 from a cordless phone, it will work just like a desk phone or a wall phone.

Cell phones (also known as wireless phones) are self-contained telephones. They work all alone: no wire needed to plug into the wall. Indeed, wireless phones don't need a house or a building, either. If you call 911 from a wireless or cell phone, the 911 operator might not know where you are. It's very important to describe where you are if you're using a cell phone.

Technology works faster than government—no surprise there—so although cell phones were getting more affordable and cheaper to buy, the government agencies in charge of 911 services were still working on the assumption that everyone was calling 911 from a phone wired up to the grid. When nobody was looking, calls to 911 from cell phones started outnumbering calls from landlines.

Now, 911 centers are starting to catch up to the technology, but there are still lots of places in the country where the call taker is not going to know where you are because the 911 center's computers don't know how to talk to the cell phone company's computers.

Indeed, if you call 911 from a cell phone, the folks who answer your call might not be in the same town you are. I live in California. Until recently in almost every town here, when you called 911 from a cell phone, the California Highway Patrol (CHP) answered the call. Once the CHP figured out which city you were in, they'd route the call to the correct 911 center.

What that means for you is that if you call 911 from a cell phone, it's important to know where you are. It's also a good idea if you're in a building to use the phone attached to the wall rather than the phone from your pocket or purse.

Even if the 911 center can pinpoint you, they might not be spot on. For instance, if you're staying in a hotel and call 911 from your cell phone, the 911 center might be able to figure out the building you're in, but they don't know what room or even what floor. You'll have to tell them.

When you call 911 from a cell phone have two pieces of information ready and right away tell whoever answers:

1. Where you are, including the town. The 911 center might not even know which town you're calling from.
2. What kind of help you need: ambulance, fire department, or police.

When I call 911 from a cell phone, as soon as a human answers I say what I want without being asked and regardless what the call taker says.

Call taker: "911. What's your emergency?"
Me: "I'm at the Fairmont Hotel in San Francisco and I need an ambulance."

Now the call taker knows which service in which city the call should be routed to. He or she is already going to be a little annoyed with me, because I didn't answer the question, but even if he or she didn't hear what I said, it's recorded and he or she can listen back if we get disconnected. Now I'm going to patiently wait for him or her to ask me some questions and the call will go on as normal.

It's really important to relay your location very clearly to the 911 call taker—I can't stress that enough. I had this important point pounded into my head while staying in a hotel in Simi Valley, California with my wife and two of my daughters. A late night knock on the door woke my wife and me out of a deep sleep at about 2:00 a.m. A pair of cops at the door asked if we would let them come in to check the room. It seems a little girl was on the phone with a 911 call taker saying she was trapped in a bathroom in that hotel.

If the little girl had called from a room phone (an option she may not have had) the 911 center would have been able to tell the cops exactly where she was. Because she called from a cell phone, the officers had to go door to door to find her. I never heard the outcome, but I hope she was okay.

Now that we've seen what's wrong with cell phones and 911, let's see what's right: Cell phones don't need to be active to reach 911. In other words, if you have a cell phone that turns on (the battery is charged) and that has a signal, it will connect to 911. You don't have to be paying for service. All you have to do is dial 911 and it will ring.

All the issues with calling 911 from a cell phone still exist if you're using a cell phone with no service contract. The 911 center still doesn't know where you are and the older the cell phone, the more likely that they can't pinpoint your location.

There's one other issue that is unique to phones with no contract: the phone doesn't have a number. You see, if the phone doesn't have a service contract, then there's no reason for it to ring, which means it won't have a number.

When you call 911 and the call taker asks you for a phone number in case you get disconnected, you won't have one. So if you get disconnected, it will be your responsibility to call 911 back.

OTHER WAYS TO CALL FOR HELP

Besides calling 911, there are other ways to get help—especially when it's not quite an emergency. Many cities around the country offer 311 service, which is intended to be an easy-to-remember number for non-emergencies. Because 311 service is not standardized, it may get you through to only a law enforcement agency—but not an ambulance—in one city, and may connect you to all services in another. Plus, 311 service is still relatively new and is only available in some places.

WHEN MEDICAL ALERT SYSTEMS GO BAD

There are a lot of medical alert systems to choose from and they're changing all the time. As the medical community sees more and more of these units, we learn more about how to get the most out of them.

We also learn how they go wrong. I think these are valuable tools, especially for seniors who choose to live alone. If you're going to have one, however, you should know what might make them malfunction. Here are a few of the ways medical alert systems can either fail or make things worse:

Telephone troubles: These systems all rely on your telephone line to call for help. They only work if you have a telephone jack to plug them into. They won't work with cell phones. Some of these systems won't work with Internet-based phones.[1]

If your telephone is off the hook when you push the button, the device won't be able to call out. To make sure the medical alert will always work, you can have someone install a *line seizure device* so the medical alert can make a call even when you have the phone off the hook on another extension.

One company refuses to offer wristband-style panic buttons because it claims that some users were unable to push the button after a stroke. Strokes can lead to one side of the body being paralyzed and apparently the users weren't able to reach the button on their wrists with their opposite hands.

The U.S. Food and Drug Administration (FDA) released a report that some users were strangulated by the panic buttons worn on a lanyard around the neck.[2] Some companies offer breakaway lanyards, whereas others claim that breakaway lanyards could come off during a fall, which would make the whole shebang pretty useless.

It's important to keep the medical alert company (or the device if it's the stand-alone kind) up to date. The operators will only know where to send help if you let them know if and when you move. They'll only be able to call friends and family if you keep their phone numbers current. It's a good idea to set aside a day every year to go over the information you have on file. Most medical alert companies will ask, but you have to make sure you let them know as soon as the information changes.

Ambulances, law enforcement agencies, and fire departments all have regular, non-emergency phone numbers listed in the phone book. Anyone can use these numbers to ask questions and arrange routine services. If you need to arrange a future trip in an ambulance, after surgery for example, you would call the non-emergency phone number to book the date and time. In most cases, non-emergency use of an ambulance is arranged through your doctor or insurance.

Many insurance or health maintenance organization (HMO) carriers also have advice lines that help you decide how to proceed when you're not sure what to do. If you think you might have a condition that needs medical attention but don't know whether you should call an ambulance, an advice line could guide you on how to proceed.

What if you can't get to the phone? As you'll see in Chapter 13, falls are the most common way for seniors to get hurt. Once on the ground, crawling to a phone might not be an option. Medical alert systems provide a way to call for help easily.

Medical alert systems come in two basic varieties: monitored or stand-alone. All systems come with a button that you carry around with you. Most of the time you wear the button on a lanyard around your neck or you can wear it strapped to your wrist like a watch.

When you push the button, the system calls for help. Monitored medical alert systems notify a live operator at a call center. The operator will talk to you through a box that looks a lot like an answering machine. If you can't answer (or you're out of range), the operator will call 911 for you. If you'd rather have a friend or relative come to your aid, the operator can call them instead.

Stand-alone systems work similarly, except that when you push the button, the box that looks like an answering machine starts making phone calls. It will call whichever telephone numbers you programmed into it. When someone answers, it will play a recorded message to let them know that you have pushed the button. These devices can be programmed to call 911, but that shouldn't be the first number that it tries.

Monitored systems provide the best service, because a live operator is going to be able to solve problems when all the folks on your list aren't answering the phone or if you need 911. The operator is a better option for most people.

On the other hand, stand-alone medical alert systems don't require a subscription. Once you buy the equipment, the system is free. It just sits there, ready to call whomever as soon as you need it to. It does require you to update it if someone on your phone list moves or changes phone numbers, but that's true even if you have a subscription to a monitored system.

Medical alert systems are great tools for seniors living alone. But just like any tool, you have to know how it works to get the best bang for your buck and what can go wrong.

The hallmark of a medical alert system is the panic button, usually worn around the neck. Most of the time, the button simply activates the system. From there, the box that's plugged into the phone line (the one that looks like an answering machine) does all the work. When the operator tries to contact you, his or her voice is going to come out of that box. To speak to him or her, you're going to be talking to the box.

If the box is too far away, on a different floor, or inside the house while you're outside, you and the operator may not be able to hear each other. Some medical alert companies offer extra boxes so you can be heard from the second floor or from the opposite side of the house. Some companies offer panic buttons with a microphone and speaker, so you can speak to the operator right from the button around your neck.

Depending on the ambulance agency, you might get charged for the response, even if the ambulance wasn't needed. In my experience, 911 calls from medical alert systems run the gamut from very serious to absolutely nothing. Sometimes we arrive to find the system has been activated completely by accident.

Some systems offer *activity monitors*. These are daily or weekly checks by the operators to make sure seniors living alone are still kicking. In theory, it's a great idea. In reality, most of the activity alarm calls we get are from seniors going on trips and not telling the alarm company. This service usually costs more money. Save your pennies; activity monitors are not worth the cost.

Getting help is about being resourceful. The best option in an emergency is 911, but it's not necessarily an emergency every time you need a little help. Having another option around—like a cell phone or a medical alert system—is always a good idea. Falling is a legitimate concern and you should have the tools to get help when you need it, even if you don't need an ambulance.

On the Internet

- www.911.gov
- www.firstaid.about.com/od/callingforhelp
- www.nena.org

3
Gearing Up

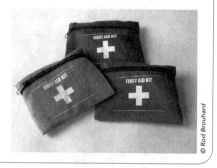

© Rod Brouhard

Whenever I talk about first aid, people always ask, "What should I keep in my first aid kit?"

First aid is really about knowing what to do and working with what you have to do it. Indeed, for most of us, first aid should be ancillary to our lives. It's for those just-in-case moments, not the focus of your days. Live life, and when you hit a bump, take care of it and get back to living.

Most people already have all the supplies they really need at home. Before we called it the *first aid kit,* we called it the *medicine cabinet,* or the *glove compartment,* or the *purse.* Indeed, I'll bet you can find at least three or four items from the list below in your home right now.

There is such a thing as being prepared, but I'm not talking about backpacking in the Himalayas. I'm talking about what you need for life's little emergencies around the house. I think you have almost everything you need already. Here's what I assume:

- *I assume you have running water.* Cuts and scrapes just need to be cleaned with water. That's it; nothing special that needs to be stored in a first aid kit. Plain tap water is what hospitals use. If it's good enough for the hospital, it's good enough for the rest of us.
- *I assume you have liquid soap.* Occasionally, if there's quite a bit of grime in those cuts, a little soap helps. Don't use bar soap because when the bar is dry, bacteria grows on it. That doesn't happen to liquid soap— you just squirt what you need out of the container and the rest of the soap stays untouched until you need it.
- *I assume you have a phone.* If it's a serious emergency, call 911. Most likely, there will be someone on the line who can tell you what to do next. Regardless of whether there's anyone to talk you through it (see Chapter 2 for more about 911), help is on the way.

Assuming you have water, soap, and a phone, you have what you need for almost anything. There're a few more items to round out your kit and you'll be set.

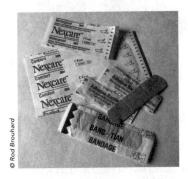

© Rod Brouhard

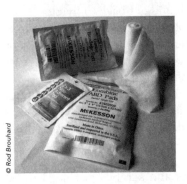

© Rod Brouhard

- *Adhesive bandages of several shapes and sizes.* These are ubiquitous with first aid. The little pad of gauze catches any blood or pus that oozes out, and by covering your cut, it heals without scabbing or scarring as badly. Knuckle bandages are hourglass-shaped bandages designed to cover battle-damaged knuckles.
- *Gauze.* Usually available in 2 × 2- or 4 × 4-inch squares, gauze is used for bigger cuts and moderate to severe bleeding. If you feel the need to dig gauze out of your first aid kit, you'll want to consider whether your wound needs stitches. You can buy roller gauze by the foot and you can roll it on to cover cuts and scrapes on delicate skin—no tape necessary. Roller gauze is also good for large injuries, such as head wounds.
- *Hand sanitizer.* Rule #1 of first aid: wash your hands. Rule #2: if you can't wash your hands, use an alcohol-based antiseptic gel on them.
- *Paper tape.* For those with delicate skin, paper tape is a must. It doesn't stick as aggressively (which means it falls off easier) and doesn't rip the skin off when you remove it. Rule of thumb: paper-thin skin gets paper tape.
- *Self-adherent bandage.* The advantage of paper tape is that it can be placed anywhere: head, chest, fingers, and so on. However, if you are able to wrap all the way around an injury—on an arm or leg, for example— self-adherent bandages are the best. They will not stick to anything but themselves.
- *Non-stick gauze pads.* There are several brands. Telfa pads are an old standby, but I like petroleum jelly gauze instead.
- *Transparent film dressing.* Anyone prone to skin tears (Chapter 17) needs to keep some of these dressings handy. Skin tears can't handle strong tape, so film dressings provide a way to treat them without causing more damage.

- *Butterfly closures*. Not every cut needs stitches. In fact, thin, delicate skin can't handle being sewn together. Butterfly closures are little strips of sterile tape (sometimes known as SteriStrips) that hold the edges of a cut together so it can heal.
- *Elastic bandages* (not the same as roller gauze). Twist an ankle or sprain a wrist? The best treatment is rest, ice, compression, and elevation (RICE). All these steps are to reduce swelling and pain. Elastic bandages take care of compression. A well-known brand of elastic bandage is the ACE Bandage.
- *Scissors*. It's really hard to take your shirt off with a broken arm or a dislocated shoulder. Likewise, it's difficult to slip your slacks off with a broken hip. Save the body part; cut the clothing off instead. Scissors are also handy for cutting roller gauze and elastic bandages down to size.
- *Tweezers*. Nothing beats a pair of tweezers for removing splinters and ticks or picking dirt out of a cut. Spend a couple of extra bucks and get a pair of good tweezers.

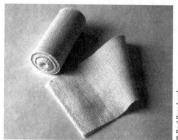

© Rod Brouhard

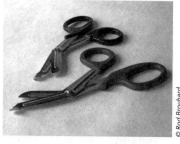

© Rod Brouhard

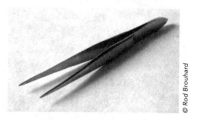

© Rod Brouhard

You may notice some things I left out, like antibiotic ointment, pain relievers, and hydrogen peroxide.

I have my reasons. First of all, putting drugs of any type in a first aid kit (including minor pain relievers and creams or ointments) is a decision you shouldn't take too lightly. First aid kits are build-'em-and-forget-'em endeavors. Putting medications in your first aid kit means the kit now has an expiration date.

How often do you open up your first aid kit and take inventory of what's in there? You will today because you just read this. Maybe you take a look when you're getting ready to go on a trip or if a big storm is coming.

Once you put medications with expiration dates in your first aid kit, you've created more work for yourself. It's not a bad idea to have some Advil or Tylenol in your kit, particularly if you're taking it on the road, but drugs won't do you any good if you let them expire in there. So plan for the medications in your first aid kit to expire and be sure to check them at least once every 6 months.

There are lots of antibiotic ointments on the market. Most have the same three antibiotics in them: neomycin, polymyxin B, and bacitracin. So many people are allergic to one or more of these antibiotics that these kinds of creams are the most common cause of allergic dermatitis (red, irritated skin) in the United States. Even more important, I don't recommend these ointments because there's no evidence that using antibiotic ointments actually prevents cuts from getting infected. Keeping cuts covered helps them heal better and keeping them moist might cut down on scarring, but as for infections, ointments don't help.

When I was a kid, my mom liked to put mercurochrome on all my cuts. Now we understand how dangerous mercury is and mercurochrome isn't available anymore. I'm lucky I didn't turn into the Mad Hatter.

Her other favorite was hydrogen peroxide, which is still widely available. You might even have some in your medicine cabinet. It's good for getting stains out (including blood stains) and cleaning up certain types of spills. It's not good, however, for cleaning open sores or cuts and scrapes.

Hydrogen peroxide is really hard on skin and muscle tissue. It causes damage that can lead to scarring. It's been used for years in surgery, but has caused bubbles in the bloodstream that led to strokes and heart attacks. And, like antibiotic ointments, hydrogen peroxide is just not necessary for preventing infections or making your injury heal faster. Remember, water is all you need.

So when you're planning or building your first aid kit, stick with dry goods. Drugs are okay, especially if you'll be traveling with your first aid kit, but plan on checking it periodically for expired medications.

SMOKE AND CARBON MONOXIDE DETECTORS

A smoke detector and a carbon monoxide detector should be included in your emergency supplies. Smoke detectors are usually permanently mounted on the ceiling (sometimes on the wall). Carbon monoxide detectors may be mounted, or they may be plugged into an electrical outlet. Some smoke detectors also detect carbon monoxide levels.

All smoke detectors are not created equal. There are two different types of smoke detectors: *ionization* and *photoelectric*. Which one you need depends on whether the fire burning in your house is slow and smoldering or big with lots of open flame. Because you won't know that until the fire actually starts, I recommend you get a smoke detector that works both ways. Different types of smoke detectors do not detect the different types of fire, so just buy a combo-style smoke alarm. If you can find one that also has a carbon monoxide detector, then you're set.

FANCY LIFESAVING GEAR

As you get a little older and technology gets more advanced, new equipment that might help you in a medical emergency becomes available. Just in the time I've been a paramedic, there have been major improvements in medical emergency equipment for the layperson. Two of the biggest improvements are automated external defibrillators (AEDs) and automatic injectors for things like epinephrine. Just because they're available, however, doesn't mean you need them.

A defibrillator is a shock box. It's the thing that delivers a jolt to your heart to get it going again after it stops beating. There are two kinds, manual and automatic, kind of like a car can have either a manual or an automatic transmission. When driving a manual transmission car, you have to know how and when to change gears. Using a manual defibrillator is the same way, so paramedics and doctors learn when and how to shock your heart.

When you drive a car with an automatic transmission, you just have to tell the car you want to drive forward and it picks the right gears for you. You still have to know how to do the rest, like steering, braking, and following the rules of the road. Using an AED is the same way. It's automated, so it will figure out when and if to shock the heart. You still have to know whether or not this is the right time to use it and how to put it on.

Automatic injectors have their place in emergencies and can certainly save lives in the right situations, but they are very specific. Epinephrine is the most common drug found in an automatic injector. The most common brand name is the EpiPen and you can see how to use one in Chapter 19. Automatic injectors are prescription medications given to you by your doctor. You should never try to use someone else's auto-injector on yourself, even if you think you have the same problem and it's the right drug. If you're wrong, it could have dire consequences. It's not a bad idea to know how to use one, especially if a family member carries one, but only use it on the person for whom it is prescribed.

I'm a believer that keeping things low-tech is the best policy. There's less to go wrong in an emergency and, just like anything else in life, you have to do the basic things first. Don't worry too much about getting fancy tools for the job. Worry instead about learning what to do in case something happens and have a plan for how to handle emergencies.

On the Internet

- firstaid.about.com/od/firstaidkits
- www.mayoclinic.com/health/first-aid-kits/FA00067

4

A Medical History of Me (That's You)

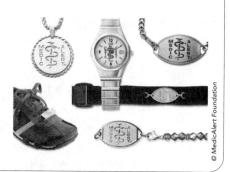

© MedicAlert Foundation

If you take more than one medication, I bet you can't write down the names of all your medications and the dosages right now without looking at the bottles. I can't remember mine, and as I write this I only take two medications. I know the names, but I'm not sure of the dosages. (I've sat here staring at the computer trying to remember the dosages of my medications for almost 5 minutes now.)

Imagine being in the worst pain you've ever felt in your entire life and having a paramedic sticking a needle in your arm while another one is putting electrocardiogram (EKG) stickers on your chest. A third rescuer is knocking over your favorite vase in the hallway while he or she is trying to get the ambulance cot closer to you.

In the middle of all this, one or more of them is firing questions at you:

"Where do you hurt?"
"What medications do you take?"
"Is there anyone else in the house?"
"What hospital do you want to go to?"
"Do you have any allergies?"
"Are you having trouble breathing?"
"When was the last time you were in the hospital?"

Do you think you'll be able to answer everything without making any mistakes? If you forget to tell the paramedic you're allergic to shellfish and he or she uses iodine on your skin, you could have an allergic reaction serious enough to kill you. If you forget to tell him or her about your heart attack last month, it could delay important treatment at the hospital later.

The trick is to write down your history. I call that the "Medical History of Me." It's your medical information, all in one place so my paramedic colleagues and I can see what types of things might be contributing to your current problem. If we're there because you're unconscious, your Medical

History of Me might tell us why. Plus, we'll take it with us to the hospital for the doctor to read.

NEED TO KNOW OR NICE TO KNOW?

Now, to put things into perspective, let me explain the difference between what is nice to know and what is really, really important.

Paramedics don't *need* to know anything about you to treat the worst possible emergencies. We are regularly called to treat people in cardiac arrest (when the heart stops beating), and we certainly can't ask them any questions. We have to go by whatever we can find, but we don't spend too much time looking. The important thing is getting blood flowing again and that's what we focus on.

When people are unconscious but the heart is working well and they are still breathing, we have more time to look around for information. If there isn't an obvious list of medicines or medical problems, we can figure it out by finding pill bottles around. Bottom line: we just don't need any information about you to treat you. The most important stuff is what we can see: sex, approximate age, injuries, and vital signs. Is your arm bent in an anatomically incorrect direction? I can treat that.

All the rest is nice to know. It's the stuff that will help us treat you faster. Are you diabetic? If we know it, we'll rule out whether that's the problem right away. If we don't know it, we'll still check your blood sugar, but maybe not at first.

We like the nice-to-know information because it makes it easier to focus our assessment in the right direction early. It gets you the care you need faster and more accurately. So having that information handy will help you get better care, but not having it won't stop you from getting the care you need.

WHAT TO INCLUDE ON THE MEDICAL HISTORY OF ME

The most important thing we need to know is your name, sex, and date of birth. This is the standard way medical folks keep track of patients. We can share information accurately if we know who we are sharing information about. We can figure out your sex, but you have to tell us your name and date of birth.

We also want to know your current medications. Statistically, if you're taking more than two medications, there is a 100% chance at least two of them are interacting in your body. That also means if you're taking more than one medication and I or my colleagues adds one to the mix by giving you a shot, it will interact with one of the medicines you're already taking. The interaction might not be serious, but it helps if we know it's coming.

Include all your daily medications—prescriptions or over-the-counter—plus supplements and vitamins. Vitamins are just medicines by a different name, and if you're taking Tylenol or Advil on a daily basis, we need to know. If you take a baby aspirin every day—whether the doctor told you to or not—tell us about it. Anything you take every day should be on that list.

In addition to medications, tell us if you have any allergies. I'm not talking about hay fever (although that's okay to know, too). I'm referring to food and drug allergies. If you can't take it or eat it, it's important. Some allergies seem harmless, but are very serious for you. If you're allergic to eggs, you can't have some antibiotics or vaccines. If you're allergic to shellfish, you probably can't tolerate iodine swabs on your skin or the dye they use for some computed tomography (CT) scans. If you don't know of any allergies, put down: "No Known Allergies." If you don't put anything on the list about allergies, we won't know if you don't have any or if you just forgot to mention them.

Lastly, we want to know about your medical history. Any diagnosis the doctor gave you is important to us, even if it seems like you don't have it anymore. If it requires medication to control it, you still have the problem; it's just being successfully treated.

I don't know how many times I've had this conversation:

Me: "Mr. Smith, do you have any medical problems?"
Mr. Smith: "Nope."
Me: "Do you take any medications?"
Mr. Smith: "Oh, yes. Several."
Me: "What do you take?"
Mr. Smith: "Oh, I take metformin and/or Glucophage to control my blood
    sugar. I take atenolol and lisinopril to control my blood pressure, and
    I take digoxin to control my irregular heartbeat."
Me: "I thought you said you don't have any medical problems."
Mr. Smith: "I don't. There's no problem as long as I take the pills."

Write it down. It matters. Besides, when the pain in your chest is so bad it makes you sweat, you're going to have a hard time remembering your medical history. Included in this chapter is a blank "Medical History of Me" form for keeping your medical information organized. Feel free to copy and use the form. It's important to keep it updated whenever things change.

A note about rare diseases: paramedics aren't going to know much about diseases that aren't very common. If you have trouble finding a doctor who's heard of your disease, you can bet good money that the paramedic who answers your 911 call is not going to know anything about that disease.

LIFE'S little
EMERGENCIES

Medical History of Me
Date Last Updated: _____

Name:	Birthday:
Allergies:	❑ No Known Allergies

Medical Conditions (Medical History)

❑ High Blood Pressure	Details: _____
❑ Heart Disease or Past Heart Attacks	_____
❑ Atrial Fibrillation/Irregular Heart Beat	_____
❑ Pacemaker	_____
❑ COPD/Asthma. Use Oxygen? ❑ Yes or ❑ No	_____
❑ Diabetes. Take insulin? ❑ Yes or ❑ No	_____
❑ Past Stroke. Weak one side? ❑ Yes or ❑ No	_____
❑ Seizures/Convulsions	_____
❑ Cancer Type? _____	_____
❑ Panic Attacks/Anxiety	_____
❑ GERD/Gastric Reflux	_____
❑ Liver Disease	_____
❑ Kidney Failure Dialysis? ❑ Yes or ❑ No	_____

Medication Name	Medication Dose	Times Medications Taken (Breakfast, Lunch, Dinner, Bedtime)

Primary Physician Name:	Phone:
Medical Insurance:	ID #:
Insurance Phone Number:	Group #:

Emergency Contact Name:	Phone:
Emergency Contact Name:	Phone:

If you have a rare disease, then you might want to put a little more information in your Medical History of Me than the name of the disease. For example, if you have *benign essential tremor*, I might not have heard of that. You should tell me some important things like where your tremors are and if you have any weakness, otherwise I might think you've had a stroke when you really haven't.

While we're talking about what information to put on your Medical History of Me, let's talk about the information you should *never* put on there: your social security number. I don't see any problem putting medical insurance information—in fact, I think it's not a bad idea. However, there is no reason anyone at the hospital or on the ambulance team needs your social security number. It's not a big deal if you give it to them (many ambulance personnel and hospitals ask for it) but you don't want a piece of paper with your name, birthday, and social security number floating around. That's a recipe for identity theft.

WHERE TO KEEP YOUR MEDICAL HISTORY OF ME

I go to senior facilities to talk to residents about emergency preparedness and they always want to know where to keep their Medical History of Me. At least one person always asks about keeping it in the refrigerator. Here's the deal: I'm not going to look in the refrigerator for your medical information.

I might look in your fridge to see if you're eating well. I might look to see if you're taking insulin (which should be stored in the fridge and would tell me that you're diabetic). If I do look in the fridge, I might see a vial with your history in it.

Then again, I might not.

Putting your information in the fridge is about as good or about as bad as putting it anywhere else in your house. There's no secret paramedic signal that tells us you've got info in the fridge. We're trained to look all over the house for clues about your medical problems and current medications. We'll probably look in the fridge, and if you put your medical information in there and make it really obvious, we might see it.

Of course, if you're awake you can say, "Look in the fridge. My medical information is in there." We should be able to find it then. You could also say, "Look on the counter" or "Look in the medicine cabinet" just as easily. It doesn't matter. Tell a family member where you keep your Medical History of Me (or give your family copies) and they can help us find it.

There are all kinds of products on the market to help you put your Medical History of Me in front of my face. Jewelry is the most common idea most people think of. In a town near me is the mother of all medical jewelry suppliers, MedicAlert. MedicAlert invented the concept. The company has a distinct logo and I'm pretty sure I've seen a picture of one of their products in every paramedic and EMT textbook I've read.

What most people don't realize is that MedicAlert is more than just the jewelry. If you look at the emblem, there's a phone number on it. MedicAlert has a call center staffed around the clock to answer that phone number, and you can make the call collect from anywhere in the world.

Here's the cool part: MedicAlert keeps all your medical information in a computer and can read it over the phone to any health care provider who calls. They'll also fax it (and probably e-mail it as well).

It's a great concept and although I must admit that paramedics constantly fail to notice the jewelry, it does help sometimes. Most paramedics aren't likely to take time out to make the phone call (some do), but hospitals use it regularly. If nothing else, it lets the hospital track down someone in your family, which should also be in the computer.

MedicAlert charges a yearly fee for keeping the medical information up to date, but like any other medical history, it's only as accurate as you make it. You have to make sure you get on the computer or make the phone call and update it. If you fail to pay your yearly fee, MedicAlert will still answer the phone and will still provide the information they have on file, but they'll also be sure to tell whoever's calling that the information is out of date.

There are lots of other medical information programs out there. Most of them try to do the same thing MedicAlert is doing, but do it cheaper. Usually, though, that just means it's not done as well. If you pay your yearly fee, MedicAlert will pester you to update stuff. Sometimes, that prodding is worth the price.

KEEP YOUR MEDICAL HISTORY OF ME LOW-TECH

The basic MedicAlert bracelet or necklace is decidedly low-tech. I like that. It doesn't take special equipment to read the bracelet (other than maybe a pair of reading glasses). It doesn't require a computer or a power source.

You may have seen some products on the market that plug into a computer. Some of them are designed to be carried on your keychain or worn around your wrist like a MedicAlert bracelet. Indeed, MedicAlert offers its own version.

Don't buy a computer-based doohickey. Nobody is going to use it. Most paramedics don't have access to a computer capable of reading those devices and the hospital doesn't want to put something like that into one of its computers for fear of a computer virus shutting down the whole operation.

Keep it low-tech. If you don't want to pay someone else to write stuff down for you (I don't blame you), then write it down yourself and keep copies handy in case you have to call an ambulance or go to the emergency room. If you travel, take copies with you.

Don't Get Scammed

Since I started covering first aid for About.com, I've heard over and over again about a company called EMT Alert. The premise is that for a few hundred bucks, EMT Alert will provide your medical information to your city's paramedic service. In most of the cases I've heard, EMT Alert claims you have to purchase its service in order to receive a response from 911.

It's not true.

There is no reason to prevent emergency responders coming out to your home unless the mother of all disasters has happened and there's just nobody left to help you. Otherwise, calling 911 is enough.

Putting It on ICE

A few years ago, there was a movement to add a special notation to the contacts in your cell phone. It was to show who you should call in case of an emergency (ICE). It was a novel idea, developed by a paramedic from the United Kingdom.

It caught on pretty well, and now there are lots of folks who put "ICE" next to their spouses' names or kids' names in their cell phones. Sounds neat, but full disclosure here: I've never looked in a cell phone for the "ICE" contact.

Never. Not once.

Some paramedics might. I'm sure the guy who thought of it looks. But I don't. I've got other things to do, like treating your life-threatening injuries. And from talking to my colleagues, they don't look much, either.

I will, however, take your cell phone to the hospital where someone is much more likely to look through it for people to call. So go ahead and put "ICE" in there, just don't be upset if the phone call comes from the hospital an hour after the car accident, rather than from the paramedic at the scene.

Your Wishes for the Worst-Case Scenario

It's that conversation you never wanted to have with your spouse or your kids: How do you want them to handle it when your ticker stops? Do you want everything done to save you? Nothing?

We're not really talking about a history anymore. Now we're talking about the future. Hopefully, we're talking about the distant future.

There's a whole lot of confusion out there about the differences in choices and what they all mean. To get started, let me give you the basics. There are three different end-of-life legal avenues you can take:

- Do not resuscitate order (DNR). This is when you talk to your doctor and she writes an order for all health care providers to follow (including paramedics), which says "don't do CPR."
- Advanced directive. This is more detailed than a DNR, but it is less official. An advanced directive tells health care providers what you want. It's something you can type up or your doctor could help you with. You can find advanced directive forms on the Internet.
- Durable power of attorney for health care. This is a legal document your lawyer makes for you. It designates someone to make medical decisions for you in case you lapse into a coma or knock your noggin hard enough to stop making sense. Choose wisely; this is the person who decides when to pull the plug.

Like the Medical History of Me, these very important documents have to be found to be followed. When someone is terminally ill and at home with a DNR, I always recommend a copy be taped to the wall above the bed. If the paramedics are called, they'll know right away what your wishes are.

Let's assume, however, that you don't have a terminal illness. Maybe you've just heard way too many horror stories of folks surviving on life support after a major stroke. Maybe you just don't want to live like that or be a burden to your children. Fair enough, but I don't recommend a DNR for that situation.

Sometimes, health care providers don't try as hard when there's a DNR. It's not something I'm proud of saying about my colleagues, but it's absolutely true.

Write up an advanced directive or a durable power of attorney for health care and let your loved ones know exactly what you want. Give copies to everyone who may need one if the time comes. That way, you get the care you need (performed with gusto) until you've decided you don't need it anymore.

ON THE INTERNET

- www.medicalert.org
- firstaid.about.com/od/Medical-History

5

Oh, What a Pill

I used to pride myself on being drug free, and then my doctor raised an eyebrow at my blood pressure. Now I have to take a couple of medications to keep it under control.

Oh! You thought I meant *the other kind* of drug free? Well, yeah, I'm that, too.

As far as I'm concerned, keeping track of my medications is pretty easy: every morning I take one of each pill. That's it, just two pills a day. I'm not organized enough to order my prescription by mail 3 months at a time, but I do use my pharmacy's website to order refills and they send me e-mail reminders when I should be getting low.

All in all, my situation is fairly simple. But what if I had more medications? What if I had to take one of my pills twice a day and the other pill three times? What if I had trouble seeing or arthritis in my fingers? The more medications and barriers there are, the more complicated it gets to take pills appropriately.

There are all kinds of methods for keeping track of your medications and pills. The easiest and most low-tech version is a piece of paper with spaces to keep track of medicine names, dosages, times, and whether you took them or not. For your convenience, we've added a form like that in this chapter. Just pull it out and fill it out (make a few copies of the blank form so you can make changes in the future). If you want, you can also go to the website http://lifes-little-emergencies.rodbrouhard.com to print out more copies of the form and find other helpful tools.

There are other tools available to help organize and dispense medication correctly. Your corner drugstore likely has a large selection of plastic organizers with little compartments for each day of the week. Some of these organizers even have multiple compartments for each day to represent morning, noon, evening, and bedtime pills.

Several of the same companies that provide medical alarm devices (see Chapter 2) also offer computerized pill dispensers that beep when it's time to take your medication. Some of those even have automatic drawers that pop out with whatever pills you need to take.

The problem with all of these solutions is that you have to do it yourself. You have to load the organizers and the dispensers. You have to fill out the medication forms and keep track of taking your pills. You have to program the fancy dispenser so it knows what time of day to open each drawer (the grandkids could probably program the dispenser, but you'll still have to load it).

No matter what kind of process you use to keep track of your medications, *you have to keep up with it*. It's the same with your Medical History of Me; only you can make sure it's updated.

There is one exception, however. If you want to pay for it, your local pharmacy may offer medication organization. You have to pick up your medications more often that way, but the pharmacist will organize your medications in a package for you. When it's time to take your pills, just pop them out of the package. It works both as an organizer and a record of what you took.

The added benefit of having your pharmacist organize your medications is that he or she will not let you take medications together that will cause a reaction. Your pharmacist will talk to you about changing your prescriptions if it looks like there will be a problem.

QUESTIONS FOR THE PHARMACIST

Pharmacists are not utilized in ways they used to be. Now that they're employees of big chain stores instead of the owner of the shop, we tend to forget how valuable of a resource they are.

When you get new medications, there are several things you should ask the pharmacist:

- Do I have to avoid certain foods or drinks when I take this medicine?
- Should I take this medicine at a certain time of day, such as morning or bedtime?
- Can I take this medicine on an empty stomach?
- Will this affect or react with other medicines I'm taking?
- Is there anything special I should know about stopping this medication?
- Is there any vitamin, supplement, or over-the-counter medication I should not take with this medicine?
- Are there any special requirements for storing this medication?

In fact, you should always ask your pharmacist what to watch out for as you add any new medication to your regimen, whether he or she is

LIFE'S little EMERGENCIES

Medication Planner

Name: —————————————— Birthday: ——————

Allergies: ——————————

	Medication Name	Amount of Medicine in Each Pill	How Many Pills to Take Each Time	Time to Take Each Dose	Notes
1					
2					
3					
4					
5					
6					
7					
8					
9					
10					

LIFE'S little EMERGENCIES

28-Day Medication Record

Name: _____ Birthday: _____

Month Start: _____ Month End: _____ Allergies: _____

Sunday	Monday	Tuesday	Wednesday	Thursday	Friday	Saturday
❑ Morning ❑ Noon ❑ Evening ❑ Bedtime	❑ Morning ❑ Noon ❑ Evening ❑ Bedtime	❑ Morning ❑ Noon ❑ Evening ❑ Bedtime	❑ Morning ❑ Noon ❑ Evening ❑ Bedtime	❑ Morning ❑ Noon ❑ Evening ❑ Bedtime	❑ Morning ❑ Noon ❑ Evening ❑ Bedtime	❑ Morning ❑ Noon ❑ Evening ❑ Bedtime
❑ Morning ❑ Noon ❑ Evening ❑ Bedtime	❑ Morning ❑ Noon ❑ Evening ❑ Bedtime	❑ Morning ❑ Noon ❑ Evening ❑ Bedtime	❑ Morning ❑ Noon ❑ Evening ❑ Bedtime	❑ Morning ❑ Noon ❑ Evening ❑ Bedtime	❑ Morning ❑ Noon ❑ Evening ❑ Bedtime	❑ Morning ❑ Noon ❑ Evening ❑ Bedtime
❑ Morning ❑ Noon ❑ Evening ❑ Bedtime	❑ Morning ❑ Noon ❑ Evening ❑ Bedtime	❑ Morning ❑ Noon ❑ Evening ❑ Bedtime	❑ Morning ❑ Noon ❑ Evening ❑ Bedtime	❑ Morning ❑ Noon ❑ Evening ❑ Bedtime	❑ Morning ❑ Noon ❑ Evening ❑ Bedtime	❑ Morning ❑ Noon ❑ Evening ❑ Bedtime
❑ Morning ❑ Noon ❑ Evening ❑ Bedtime	❑ Morning ❑ Noon ❑ Evening ❑ Bedtime	❑ Morning ❑ Noon ❑ Evening ❑ Bedtime	❑ Morning ❑ Noon ❑ Evening ❑ Bedtime	❑ Morning ❑ Noon ❑ Evening ❑ Bedtime	❑ Morning ❑ Noon ❑ Evening ❑ Bedtime	❑ Morning ❑ Noon ❑ Evening ❑ Bedtime

organizing them for you or not. Always fill every prescription through the same pharmacy, whether you get the prescription from your primary doctor, the emergency department doctor, or your heart surgeon. Those doctors talk to each other, but not all the time, and rarely about your medications. One doctor could prescribe a medicine that interacts in a dangerous way with something the other doctor gave you.

When you always fill your prescriptions at the same pharmacy, the pharmacist—or more likely the pharmacist's computer—will notice if the new medication will interact poorly with one you're already taking. We all know how well-laid plans sometimes do not work out, so even if you have diligently filled your prescriptions at the same pharmacy for the last 30 years, mistakes do happen.

STORING MEDICATIONS

When I go to a house on a 911 call, sometimes the only window I have into the patient's medical history is the medicine cabinet. I know if I see lisinopril that the patient has high blood pressure and if I see metformin, he or she has diabetes.

I can't see that when the labels are missing. I also can't tell if my patient's been compliant with his or her medications, taking as many as he or she is supposed to. If you transfer your medications into another container—pill organizer or something else—it's vitally important to write down what's in there, the dose per pill, when it was purchased, how many pills there were, and how many are taken every day.

If you get a refill, don't mix the pills from the old bottle in with the new bottle. Use up the old bottle of pills first, and then start with the new. That way, when I show up to your house on a 911 call I can look at the date on the prescription bottle and tell how many pills there should be in there.

EVEN IF THE COPS ARE POUNDING ON THE DOOR, DON'T FLUSH THE DRUGS

If you need to rid yourself of an unfinished bottle of pills, prescription or otherwise, never flush them down the toilet. Sending medications down the drain just releases them into the water supply, which affects everyone else. If we all dumped our pain pills in the commode, we'd all eventually get high from the tap water.

If you have leftover pills from a prescription or an over-the-counter bottle, take it back to the pharmacy. The drugstore will properly dispose of your unused medications (and no, they won't just put them in someone else's bottle).

STOPPING A DRUG CAN BE AS DANGEROUS AS STARTING ONE

Some of the medications your doctor prescribes are intended to be taken together. One of the most common combinations that comes to mind is potassium taken with furosemide (Lasix). Furosemide is a diuretic—otherwise known as a "water pill"—that is used to get rid of excess fluid in the body. Most of the time, furosemide is used to treat congestive heart failure.

Along with fluid, furosemide flushes potassium out of the body in pretty large amounts. We need potassium to make our muscles and nerves work correctly. Most importantly, we need potassium to make the cells of the heart work correctly—cells with similarities to both muscles and nerves.

VIAGRA OR NITRO? IT MIGHT BE A HARD CHOICE

I think the most deadly medication reactions aren't those that happen between two medications you take every day. Those are the types of interactions the pharmacist catches and fixes. Much more dangerous are the reactions that happen when one or both of the medications are only taken once in a while.

The most deadly reaction of this type that surfaced in the last few years was the combination of nitrates (nitroglycerin is the most common) and erectile dysfunction drugs like Viagra. Viagra started out as a cardiac drug, meant to augment or replace nitrates by doing something very similar for the heart's blood flow.

During clinical testing of Viagra, researchers discovered that this new cardiac drug had a really nifty side effect—at least for the men in the study. They promptly stopped the study and repurposed Viagra for a condition that wouldn't need to be treated every day—at least for most guys.

When Viagra hit the shelves for public consumption, a big issue was uncovered (sorry, couldn't resist): when mixed with nitrates, Viagra can cause a dangerous—sometimes fatal—loss of blood pressure. There were a few deaths reported and now the FDA strongly recommends against taking nitrates if you've taken a medication for erectile dysfunction in the last 36 hours.

If you get too low in potassium, your heart gets too weak to pump blood and you die. If you have too much potassium, your heart gets too excited to pump—and you die. Either way, the outcome is for the birds.

Many patients who take furosemide don't like the way it makes them pee (that's what it's supposed to do). When they get fed up with taking the water pill, they stop taking it but still take their potassium. Unfortunately, that may lead to a really high potassium level.

Some folks take blood pressure medication that can't be stopped all at once (ACE inhibitors and beta blockers are two classes like that). Anti-seizure medications also should never be stopped suddenly without a doctor's supervision. Stopping an antiseizure drug too quickly can result in seizures.

There are lots of medications that can't be stopped suddenly or need to be taken with other drugs, which means stopping both or neither one.

COMMON SIDE EFFECTS FOR DRUGS YOU MIGHT BE TAKING

There are some side effects for certain classes of medications that may affect you:

- *Opioid Pain Medications:* Opioid pain medications are made from opium (or a man-made version of it). That's the same stuff that heroin comes from. Opioids do two things to almost everyone (besides fix your pain): give you tiny pupils (the black part in the middle of your eye) and cause constipation. They're also highly addicting and can cause shallow breathing—or no breathing at all—if you take too much.
- *Diuretics (Water Pills):* Diuretics are used to get rid of excess fluid, but sometimes they can lead to dehydration. It's important to let your doctor know if you've been getting dizzy when you stand up, or if you're feeling weak or fatigued. Some diuretics—like Lasix—can suck potassium out of your bloodstream (see previous pages).
- *ACE Inhibitors:* These are blood pressure drugs that can cause skin rashes, hacking coughs and, oddly, loss of taste.
- *Beta Blockers:* Also blood pressure drugs that can trigger depression, impotence (did I mention depression?), cold hands, cold feet, insomnia, or a slow heartbeat. Beta blockers also mess with your ability to process blood sugar, so if you're a diabetic, you should be closely monitored while taking any of these medications.

DON'T DRUG AND DRIVE

I know I promised not to be too preachy at the beginning of this book and I'm going to stick to that. I don't think it's any of my business how you live your life. If you want to have an adult beverage or a smoke, I'm not going to tell you that you're making a mistake (although I will be honest about how it will affect your health).

I don't care how you treat your own body, but this time it isn't about you.

Many years ago, it was perfectly okay to hop in a car after a night of drinking and carrying-on. Indeed, you were unlikely to get so much as a ticket from the cops if you even got pulled over. If you were drunk enough, they might haul you down to the pokey to sleep it off.

Today we know that driving while intoxicated is a huge mistake. You can't concentrate. Your reactions are slower and your decision making is impaired. Driving under the influence causes accidents, which kill or significantly injure someone in the United States about every 20 minutes.

For some reason, although we've tightened up our belief that driving drunk is a crime and a really bad idea, we've somehow ignored the role that medications play in car crashes. There are warnings on bottles of prescriptions that tell you when you should not drive a car:

"Use Caution When Operating Machinery"

"May Cause Drowsiness"

"Alcohol May Intensify This Effect"

These are indicators that getting behind the wheel when taking these medications is as dangerous as drinking and driving—and in some cases even more so. Heed the labels. When a medication warning says not to operate machinery or that you may feel drowsy, don't drive. Have someone else take control of the wheel. It's not worth your life or someone else's.

- *Calcium Channel Blockers:* These are also blood pressure meds good for heart palpitations, constipation, fatigue, swollen ankles (which you could be taking a diuretic for), or headache. All the blood pressure medications, including the diuretics, can lead to dizziness.
- *Antibiotics:* Many people don't realize that antibiotics can lead to diarrhea and upset stomach. Sometimes they cause vomiting. Antibiotics can also cause allergic reactions.

- *Phenothiazines:* These medications are used as antihistamines, anti-nausea medications, sleep aids, and to treat mental health conditions. There is a relatively common reaction to phenothiazines known as extrapyramidal symptoms (EPS). One of the most common types of EPS is dystonia, a cramping of one side of the neck and one shoulder, along with a swollen tongue. Benadryl (diphenhydramine) will usually make the reaction go away.
- *Nonsteroidal Anti-Inflammatory Drugs (NSAIDs):* Aspirin is by far the oldest and most well known of all NSAIDs, but ibuprofen (Advil or Motrin) is quickly catching up. These drugs can upset the stomach lining and even cause bleeding.

ON THE INTERNET

- www.aarp.org/health/health_tools

II
Saving Lives

6

Your Own Mask First

E mergencies have a way of bringing out the best in some people and the worst in others. Sometimes, they can bring out both at the same time in the same person. We can let our desire to help someone overwhelm our own protective instincts.

When you fly in an airplane, the flight attendant's briefing always says to put on your own oxygen mask first, before helping someone else. That's important advice in any medical emergency. Take care of yourself first.

EMTs and paramedics are often asked why we don't run at the scene of an emergency. Actors on TV pretending to be paramedics and EMTs always run, so why don't we?

The answer is twofold. First, we are supposed to be in control. Emergency responders know the importance of getting to the patient's side safely and in control. When you call 911, you want me to show up with an ambulance, some fancy medical equipment, a team of well-trained responders, and an air of confidence. You want to feel like we have the situation under control and that you will be fine.

I don't seem so confident when I'm sucking wind because I've sprinted up your driveway.

The other reason is that we might get hurt. If I'm jogging across your front lawn and step in a gopher hole (this is just an example; I'm not suggesting you have gophers), I might twist an ankle. Then what? If I'm hurt, who takes care of you? At that point not only do I have to call out another ambulance for you but I will also have to figure out what to do with myself.

Whenever we arrive at the scene of an emergency, there are two types of family members or friends with whom we're going to interact. Either they will be calm and helpful or anxious and interfering. As you can imagine, paramedics prefer calm and helpful. That doesn't mean they're not scared for their loved one; it just means they're keeping their emotions in check in order to facilitate good care.

When you are alone and helping someone in need, you'll be much more successful if you can do the same thing we do: slow down and move deliberately. My wife—an EMT and occasional work partner of mine—absolutely hates the way I bring home my work. She sometimes wants me to move quickly and appear excited, but two decades on emergency scenes has washed that ability out of me.

I have found that moving slower and more deliberately leads to fewer mistakes being made and it makes the other folks at the scene calmer as well. Indeed, when people are yelling over each other, I speak quieter. Others will tone it down just to be able to hear me.

The other thing we don't do is take unnecessary risks. My job can be dangerous. Being a firefighter is a little more dangerous and being a police officer is even more so. We adopt certain risks just by being in the places we go, but we train regularly to handle those situations as safely as possible. The number one way to avoid getting really hurt is to stay on the script. Whenever possible, we don't wing it.

Despite that, there are times when we have to do things that are a little more dangerous to help the folks who've called us out. Maybe we have to climb onto a freeway overpass or into an overturned truck. Whatever it is, when we do take on additional risk, we try to do it as safely as possible.

I want you to do the same thing. When training folks to do CPR, one of the questions we always hear is: How long do I do CPR before I stop? There are three answers to that question:

1. When the patient wakes up (the best outcome)
2. When a rescuer or doctor tells you to stop
3. When you just can't do it any longer

Answer #3 always encourages a little discussion among the students. When can't I do it any longer? An obvious answer is when you're exhausted. If you physically can't push the chest anymore, you just have to stop. It's physics.

But there are other situations. If it's not safe to continue CPR, you should stop. An example I always used to tell my students is about two friends skiing. One of them suffers cardiac arrest and the other starts CPR. The rescuing friend tries and tries until he's just physically exhausted and can't go on. Then the rescuing friend dies of exposure because he's too exhausted to find shelter.

In that example, it makes sense for the rescuing friend to stop earlier and take care of himself. His selflessness, while honorable, ultimately led to two deaths instead of one. (Remember, this is just a story.)

How much you are willing to do for someone—and how much danger you are willing to face—is a deeply personal decision. There are lots of variables, including how well you know the person and how much help he or she needs. I don't want to tell you how to act, but I do want any decisions you make to be done as safely as possible, even if you're willing to take risks.

Emergencies need quick action by definition. There may be a life—or lives—at stake. Despite the direness of the situation, you don't have to feel or act desperate. Read through the sections of this book on preparation and on lifesaving techniques. Being prepared will be your best protection from making a mistake or getting hurt yourself.

Like the flight attendant says, put your own mask on first.

On the Internet

• firstaid.about.com/od/firstaidbasics/qt/06_leadership.htm

7

Mighty Neighborly of You

E veryone feels the need to reach out to another person in need, be it a neighbor, a friend, or a total stranger. That feeling could be overwhelming when it appears the person in need is going to die without help. It could be an immediate emergency, such as a child running into a busy street after a ball, or a slower, but no less dire need, like a family member in deteriorating health.

Such a strong feeling of compassion can lead us to impose our help on someone who may not want it. It's hard to imagine that someone in a medical emergency would not want help. If you were in the same situation, wouldn't you want any help you could get?

Indeed, the medical community assumes this very same thing. If you cannot communicate for whatever reason, the medical community is compelled to provide any lifesaving measures—at least until you can communicate again.

The reason this matters is because of *consent*, the medical word for permission to treat. Each of us is the master of his or her own body. No one has permission to lay a hand on you unless you give it to him or her. When you're unable to communicate and in need of emergency medical treatment, medical folks assume we have that permission.

When you're awake and capable of communicating, however, the game changes. No one—not even a doctor—can do any sort of treatment, lifesaving or otherwise, without you saying it's okay.

For as long as I've worked on an ambulance team, there have been neighbors and family members at the homes and bedsides of my patients. The motivations of these well-wishers and patient advocates are rarely in question. What is rare is the loved one who understands when the ambulance drives away from the house empty because the patient had the right to refuse care.

I can't count the number of times I've been at the scene of a senior patient, living alone, whose neighbor has come to the house after the senior has taken a fall. The patient just wanted a little help getting off the floor, but the compassionate neighbor, uncomfortable with the idea of emergency responders leaving the patient at home, insists we take his or her friend to be checked out.

I doubt I need to tell any reader the realities of life today. Medical care is expensive and intrusive. You have the right to decide when, where, and if you receive care. Likewise, despite how uncomfortable it might make you feel, your neighbor has the same right to choose—and to refuse.

In Chapter 4 we talked about advanced directives and end-of-life decisions. The urge to help your neighbor is so strong that if that's *not* what someone wants, he or she has to write it down in advance.

CAN YOU EVER FORCE SOMEONE TO GET HELP?

As a parent, I've seen my kids make plenty of decisions I would call mistakes—especially as adults. As a paramedic, I've seen my patients make plenty more. Sometimes, the mistake is not getting care when you need it. I've been asked by many concerned families and friends: "Can't you just make them go?"

The quick answer is no. If you have the mental capacity to understand the decision, you have the right to refuse medical care. However, there are exceptions. When a person is a danger to him- or herself (suicidal thoughts) or a danger to others (homicidal thoughts), a physician or law enforcement officer can step in and require him or her to get help.

There is one other time when a person can be seen against his or her will, and that is when he or she is gravely disabled. Unfortunately for those of us in the business of helping people, there's not a standard definition of *gravely disabled*. Consequently, folks are rarely forced to seek medical care for this reason (besides, if you're gravely disabled, you probably don't have the mental capacity to refuse, anyway).

All this neighborly love and concern is wonderful for your community, but please don't let it get in the way of a person's autonomy. If your neighbor doesn't want help, he or she shouldn't have to take it. If your neighbor is unconscious and can't communicate with you, you can assume he or she would ask for help if he or she could. Respect for a person's right to make decisions—that's what consent is all about.

No Good Deed Goes Unpunished

Almost as strong as our desire to help one another is the fear of being sued if we do. Who wants to pull a friend out of a burning car just to be blamed for the friend becoming paralyzed?[3]

Good Samaritan protections have been around for a very long time, and are intended to protect those who help others out of the kindness of their hearts. These protections weren't always laws, but started instead as legal tenets throughout the courts.

MUST I HELP AS A GOOD SAMARITAN?

People regularly tell me they never want to get a CPR certification because they don't want to be forced to help a stranger. The thought is that if you have a CPR card in your wallet, then you're bound to help, whether you want to or not. In 49 states, that's not the case.

Good Samaritan laws are mostly there to protect people who act out of their own kindness. The laws are intended to keep us from being punished for trying to be nice. There's a version of the Good Samaritan law in every state and all but one of them say pretty much the same thing. As long as you help without expecting anything in return, you are protected from liability unless you do something really, really bad.

Vermont is the one exception to the rule. In Vermont, you have to help your fellow Vermonter, whether you want to or not. If you don't help, you could be fined. Because the statute says you have to help, I recommend getting some CPR training, just in case.

Indeed, knowing CPR and first aid training is never a bad thing and neither is helping your neighbor. So don't be afraid of helping, wherever you are.

Having Good Samaritan protection through the courts is one thing, but Good Samaritan *laws* help to keep you out of court in the first place. The context of Good Samaritan laws differs from state to state, but generally they provide a way for rescuers to get the courts to dismiss a lawsuit before it really gets started.

Good Samaritan laws only protect rescuers (or would-be rescuers) who don't expect any reward. If you're getting paid or expect to get a reward for helping, you aren't a Good Samaritan. Sometimes, accepting a reward after helping—even if you didn't expect it—can cancel out any Good Samaritan protection.

As long as you are acting in the best interests of the person you are helping, without expecting anything in return, Good Samaritan laws should protect you. So be neighborly.

On the Internet

- firstaid.about.com/od/medicallegal

8

Doing CPR

Quick Decisions

| Can you wake the person? | NO | **CALL 911** |

| Is the person breathing? | NO | Start CPR: Push in the middle of the chest about two times a second |

YES

| After 911 is called, make sure the door is unlocked | | Watch for breathing |

C PR should be done on any person who will not wake up and is not breathing normally: adult, child, or infant.

ADULT CPR

Here are the steps to do CPR on an adult:

1. *Try to wake the person.* Shake the shoulders and shout his or her name. If he or she won't wake up, go to step 2.
2. *Call 911.* If the person will not wake up, call 911 immediately. If the 911 operator tells you what to do next, ignore the rest of this chapter and do what he or she tells you to do.
3. *If the person is not breathing, start pushing on the chest.* If the person isn't breathing or is only gasping, put your hands in the center of the chest, right on the breastbone, and push straight down at least 2 inches. Push at least 100 times per minute—about two pushes per second.
4. *If you've been trained to give rescue breaths and you feel comfortable doing it, then give rescue breaths.* After 30 pushes on the chest, you can give two rescue breaths if you feel

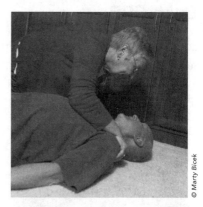

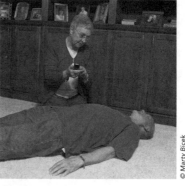

53

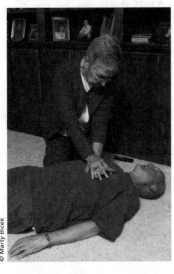

© Marty Bicek

comfortable doing so. If you've never been trained how or you just don't feel comfortable doing it, then just keep pushing on the chest hard and fast.

5. *Keep going until help arrives or the person wakes up.* If you are doing chest pushes and rescue breaths, then keep doing 30 chest pushes followed by two rescue breaths. Try not to stop doing chest pushes for more than 10 seconds at any time. If you are doing only chest pushes, then just keep pushing at least 2 inches deep and at least 100 times per minute.

CHILD CPR

CPR for infants and children is a little different than for adults. Child CPR is for kids that haven't reached puberty yet. If you have a big kid and aren't sure which kind of CPR to do, then do adult CPR. Here are the steps for child CPR:

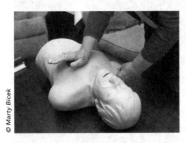

© Marty Bicek

1. *Try to wake the child.* Shake the shoulders and shout his or her name. If he or she won't wake up, go to step 2.

2. *If the child isn't breathing, start CPR now (step 3).* If someone is there with you, have that person call 911. If the 911 operator tells you what to do next, ignore the rest of this chapter and do what he or she tells you to do. If you're alone, call 911 after doing CPR for 2 minutes.

3. *Push on the chest.* If the child isn't breathing or is only gasping, put your hands in the center of the chest right on the breastbone and push down one-third of the way through the chest (about 2 inches). Push at least 100 times per minute—about two pushes per second.

4. *If you've been trained to give rescue breaths and you feel comfortable doing it, then give rescue breaths.* After 30 pushes on the chest, you can give two rescue breaths if you feel comfortable doing so. If you've never been trained how or you just don't feel comfortable doing it, then just keep pushing on the chest hard and fast.

5. *After 2 minutes, call 911 if they haven't been called already.* If you are by yourself, call 911 after 2 minutes of CPR. If someone else is there, then don't wait—call 911 while CPR is happening.

6. *Keep going until help arrives or the child wakes up.* If you are doing chest pushes and rescue breaths, then keep doing 30 chest pushes followed by two rescue breaths. Try not to stop doing chest pushes for more than 10 seconds at any time. If you are doing only chest pushes, then just keep pushing at least one-third of the way into the chest (about 2 inches deep) and at least 100 times per minute.

CPR ON A ZIPPER

Open heart surgery scars are pretty spectacular to look at. They're bold lines of scar tissue running right down the center of the chest along the breastbone. Right after surgery they're angry and red. Eventually the redness fades but the scar is always there as a reminder.

If you or your spouse has one, you know what I mean.

In the ambulance and in the hospital, we call this type of scar a *zipper.* When we see one we know the patient has had some sort of open heart surgery (valve replacements and coronary artery bypass surgeries are the most common). It looks even more like a zipper when the patient has just come out of surgery, with stitches or staples running the length of the whole incision like teeth on your favorite ski jacket.

If you are confronted with one of these scars as you're about to do CPR you may wonder: *What should I do?*

Do CPR just like normal.

The alternative to doing CPR is not doing CPR and that only has one outcome: death. It might feel weird pushing on a chest with a zipper — especially a fresh one — but it's the only way to help someone with cardiac arrest. Push hard and push fast, zipper or not.

INFANT CPR

Infant CPR is for babies younger than one year. Older kids get child CPR. Here are the steps for infant CPR:

1. *Try to wake the baby.* Flick the baby's feet (babies hate that) and shout his or her name. If he or she won't wake up, go to step 2.

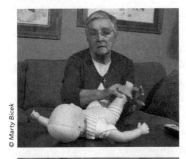

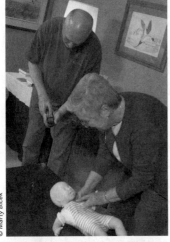

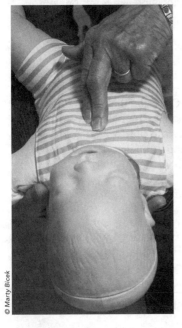

2. *If the baby isn't breathing, start CPR now (step 3).* If someone is there with you, have that person call 911. If the 911 operator tells you what to do next, ignore the rest of this chapter and do what he or she tells you to do. If you're alone, call 911 after doing CPR for 2 minutes.

3. *Push on the chest.* If the baby isn't breathing or is only gasping, put your fingers in the center of the chest right on the breastbone and push down one-third of the way through the chest (about 1½ inches). Push at least 100 times per minute—about two pushes per second.

4. *If you've been trained to give rescue breaths and you feel comfortable doing it, then give rescue breaths.* After 30 pushes on the chest, you can give two rescue breaths if you feel comfortable doing so. If you've never been trained how or you just don't feel comfortable doing it, then just keep pushing on the chest hard and fast.

5. *After 2 minutes, call 911 if it hasn't happened already.* If you are by yourself, call 911 after 2 minutes of CPR. If someone else is there, then don't wait—call 911 while CPR is happening.

6. *Keep going until help arrives or the baby wakes up.* If you are doing chest pushes and rescue breaths, then keep doing 30 chest pushes followed by two rescue breaths. Try not to stop doing chest pushes for more than 10 seconds at any time. If you are doing only chest pushes, then just keep pushing at least one-third of the way into the chest (about 1½ inches deep) and at least 100 times per minute.

CPR Training

If you got this far in this chapter, then you aren't currently pumping on anyone's chest. You're reading this because you want to know what to do in case of an emergency. Don't rely on CPR steps in a book: you should learn CPR in person.

CPR is the most basic of all medical training. It's a step-by-step, do-it-yourself process that requires very little knowledge and very little assessment. CPR is also the most important medical training anyone will ever get. Every paramedic, firefighter, nurse, doctor, dentist, police officer, physician's assistant, respiratory therapist, surgeon, and any other medical person must be trained in CPR. It's the foundation that almost all medical training builds upon. The version we learn is not that much different than the version that you will learn. CPR might be basic but, as in everything in life, the basic foundation is the most important.

Don't worry about getting certified in CPR; worry about learning to do it right. Stay away from online classes because you can't learn to do CPR on the Internet. CPR is a physical skill that gets better with practice and feedback.

On the Internet

- www.heart.org/cpr
- www.redcross.org/cpr

9

All Choked Up

Quick Decisions

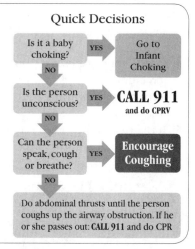

Is it a baby choking? — **YES** → Go to Infant Choking

NO

Is the person unconscious? — **YES** → **CALL 911** and do CPRV

NO

Can the person speak, cough or breathe? — **YES** → **Encourage Coughing**

NO

Do abdominal thrusts until the person coughs up the airway obstruction. If he or she passes out: **CALL 911** and do CPR

When we're talking about choking, we're talking about something stuck in the windpipe (trachea). Choking is also known as having an *airway obstruction*, which can be anything from a marble your grandson was sucking on to the piece of steak your spouse didn't chew quite well enough.

There are a couple different ways to help someone who is choking and two things to remember:

1. Don't put anything in the person's mouth to try to pry out the airway obstruction. You can do a lot of damage to the throat and windpipe that way.
2. *Anyone who is coughing or speaking is breathing, at least a little.* Some air is better than no air. Barring putting things down the throat to pry it out, whatever you can do to encourage the airway obstruction to come out is fair game—even slapping the person on the back.

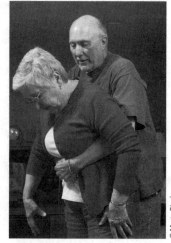

© Marty Bicek

When someone who is choking can't cough or speak anymore, he or she isn't breathing anymore. At that point, time is critical. You need to get the airway obstruction out *now*. Here are the steps to remove an airway obstruction from any person other than a baby (see further instructions for infants), that *cannot* speak or cough:

1. Stand behind him or her and wrap your arms around as if to give a hug.
2. Make a fist with one hand and place it just above his or her belly button.

3. Cover your fist with your other hand and thrust inward and upward forcefully.
4. Repeat thrusts until the person is able to breathe again or becomes unconscious.
5. If the person becomes unconscious, call 911 and begin adult CPR if he or she is an adult and child CPR if the child hasn't hit puberty yet.

Quick Decisions

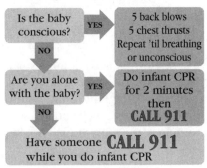

Baby Steps

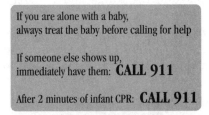

If you are alone with a baby, always treat the baby before calling for help

If someone else shows up, immediately have them: **CALL 911**

After 2 minutes of infant CPR: **CALL 911**

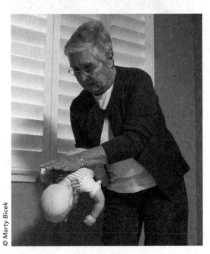

© Marty Bicek

INFANT CHOKING

Babies aren't yet built quite the same as those who are older. Their windpipes aren't as stiff and they love to put things in their mouths. Babies can handle a lot, but once there's an airway obstruction, you have only a few minutes to get it out.

Technically, an infant is any baby younger than a year old, but if you have a small baby that's maybe a few months older than a year, he or she can still be treated as an infant. The point is to get the airway obstruction out quickly. Here are the steps:

1. If someone else is with you, have them call 911 while you try to help the baby. If not, help the baby before calling 911.
2. If the baby isn't awake, do infant CPR as described in Chapter 8. After 2 minutes of infant CPR, call 911 if nobody has called already.
3. If the baby is still awake but choking: Hold the baby on your knee with his or her head down at an angle—support the baby's head and don't let it dangle. Strike him or her five times on the back with the heel of your hand, right between the shoulder blades.

4. If the baby's still choking, roll him or her onto his or her back, keeping the head low. With two fingers on his or her breastbone between the nipples, give the baby five chest thrusts, pushing the chest about one-third of the way in.

5. Repeat steps 3 and 4 until the baby starts breathing again (he or she will probably cry) or until he or she passes out. If the baby passes out, start infant CPR described in Chapter 8. After 2 minutes of infant CPR, call 911 if nobody has called already.

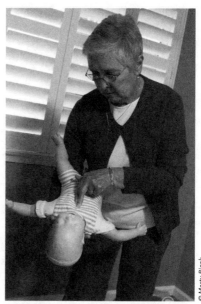

Whenever you must give a child CPR or get an airway obstruction out, have someone else call 911 while you take care of the child. If you're alone, take care of the child first and then call 911. Infants and children don't last as long without breathing as adults do. It's very important to try to get them breathing again right away, before calling 911.

ON THE INTERNET

- www.heart.org/cpr
- www.redcross.org/cpr

10

Controlling Bleeding

Bleeding Steps

1. Put pressure on the cut

2. Raise the cut above the heart

3. If the cut doesn't stop bleeding after 10 minutes: **CALL 911**

Whether blood is oozing out slowly or squirting across the room in spurts, it can almost always be controlled with pressure and time. There are two steps to controlling bleeding:

1. Hold pressure on the cut or wound
2. Raise the wound above the heart, if possible

Tourniquets should rarely be used outside of some pretty intense situations. The only reason to use a tourniquet is if you need both hands and it's going to be a while before you can get help.

TOURNIQUETS WORK GREAT: IN COMBAT

Tourniquets are constricting bands that wrap around legs or arms to help control bleeding. They're very common in the military and are used regularly on the battlefield. Tourniquets have been around since Napoleon's day and other than being modernized for quick deployment, they really haven't changed much.

Tourniquets work; there's no denying that. They stop blood flow and that stops bleeding. Once a tourniquet is applied, nobody has to hold pressure on the wound anymore. That's perfect in combat where the fighting isn't going to stop just because someone is bleeding.

The main issue with tourniquets is that they sometimes cause extra damage, especially if they're left on too long. It's a risk we don't need to take unless something is preventing us from holding pressure on the cut (like the fact that someone is shooting at us). At home—with telephones, 911, and ambulances—there's just no reason to use a tourniquet. They don't necessarily work better than pressure; they're just hands-free.

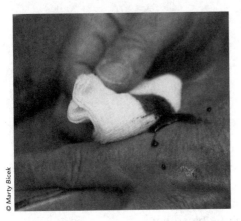

© Marty Bicek

You don't need anything in your hand to hold pressure on a wound, but it actually helps to have a bit of gauze or cloth to hold pressure. As blood soaks into the cloth or the gauze pad, it is trapped and stops moving, allowing platelets to do their job.

As you can probably imagine, holding a dirty piece of cloth up to an open wound is a recipe for infection. Using a sterile piece of gauze is ideal, but if that's not available, then at least try to use a clean cloth. You'll have to hold pressure on a bleeding wound for at least 10 minutes. Depending on how bad the bleeding is, you might have to hold pressure much longer than that.

When holding pressure on a cut, the cloth or gauze might soak through. If that happens, *do not* remove the soaked gauze or cloth. If you remove it, you'll pull all those platelets apart and open the wound up again. Instead, put a new, clean piece of gauze or cloth over the soaked one and keep holding pressure. Also, if you haven't called 911, blood soaking through the gauze or cloth is a good reason to do so.

HOW BLEEDING STOPS

Here's an old ambulance joke: All bleeding stops—eventually.

Blood is made of several ingredients: salt water (plasma), white blood cells for fighting infections, red blood cells for carrying oxygen, and platelets to help the blood clot together when necessary. Those platelets help the body control bleeding by making the blood stick together and plug leaks. When I was a kid and couldn't afford to have my car fixed, I used a product that works just like platelets do to plug leaks in my radiator.

The trick to make blood clot and stop bleeding is to trap it in place for a few minutes. The best way to do that is to put pressure on the cut. The slower blood flows, the easier it will be to trap. One thing that might help slow blood flow is gravity, so elevating a cut above the heart may slow it down. Some cuts you just can't do anything about (like cuts on the belly or the back).

Bloody Noses

Bloody noses can affect adults as well as kids. If you're taking blood thinners, bloody noses can sometimes come on suddenly without warning. When the grandkids get nosebleeds it's not that big of a deal, but when adults get them it can be very serious.

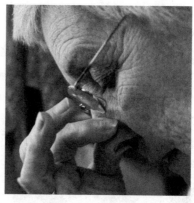

© Marty Bicek

Here are the steps to stop a nosebleed for kids or adults:

1. *Lean forward.* There's a tendency to lean back with a bloody nose to protect your favorite blouse. That's a bad idea. Blood is still flowing if you lean back; it's just going down the back of your throat instead of dripping down your shirt. You could choke on the blood. If you swallow the blood, it might irritate the lining of your stomach and cause you to vomit, which would still ruin your blouse.

2. *Pinch the nose just below the bony part.* You're trying to squish the blood vessels in your nose, not trap blood in there. If you pinch it correctly, you will still be able to breathe through your nose, but the blood will stop flowing. When that happens, you're in the right spot. Hold it for at least 5 minutes.

3. When 5 minutes are up, you can let go and see what happens. If you let go before 5 minutes, find the right spot to pinch again and start the clock over. If after 5 minutes the bleeding hasn't stopped, pinch it again, for 10 minutes this time. Remember, if you let go early, start the clock over again.

4. If a nosebleed doesn't stop after the second try, it's time to go to the emergency department. Obviously, have someone else drive you (you can't drive and hold pressure on your nose at the same time). If you're alone, you'll need to call 911.

There are a few other things you can try to help stop a bloody nose. One of which is to place ice on the nose which will cause the arteries to squeeze shut (they don't like the cold). Use ice and pressure at the same time.

If you get a nosebleed to stop, *don't blow your nose!* Blowing your nose might break any clots loose and start the whole thing over again. Let your nose heal for an hour or so before you clear it out. And whatever you do, don't pick it.

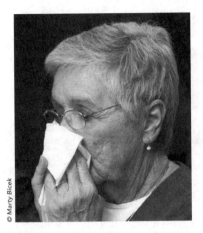

© Marty Bicek

The most common cause of bloody noses is what's known in the medical field as *digital trauma*. In other words: picking your nose. It's worse in dry air when the inside of your nose gets dried out. Sometimes, however, a nosebleed that occurs spontaneously could be a sign of extremely high blood pressure or too many blood thinners. Call your doctor if you get a bloody nose and you weren't picking it.

If your nose starts bleeding after a thump on the head, call 911. Bleeding or clear fluid coming from the nose after hitting your head could be a sign of a skull fracture (see Chapter 14).

SHOCK

The word "shock" has three meanings in first aid:

1. A jolt of electricity given to help the heart get started again when it stops suddenly. We use a device called a *defibrillator* for this.
2. That emotional state folks get into when they're traumatized: "He's *in shock* after hearing of a terrible loss."
3. The medical condition *shock* is when the brain and certain other fragile organs (kidneys and nerve cells, to name a couple) can't get enough blood to stay functioning.

Shock is a life-threatening condition. When we're injured, our bodies will reroute blood flow to protect the brain and increase how fast and how hard our hearts beat to increase the blood flow. As blood flows faster through the lungs, we also start to breathe faster to keep up.

Since blood is pulled away from our skin and toward the middle of our bodies and brains, we get pale. Regardless how dark your skin is, some of your color comes from the red blood flowing just below the surface of your skin. When it's not there, you look pale or gray. On top of all that, the adrenaline rush that comes with shock makes us sweat.

All put together, people who are severely bleeding that are going into shock will be sweating, have pale and cool skin, and be breathing fast. If all that isn't getting the brain the blood it needs, they will also be dizzy, confused, or unconscious.

SEVERE BLEEDING AND SHOCK

Severe bleeding can lead to a condition called shock if it's not controlled. Shock is a life-threatening condition that comes from too much blood loss. If you see the signs of shock, call 911 immediately:

Besides calling 911, the most important treatment for shock is to *stop the bleeding.* Once bleeding has stopped, you can cover the person with a blanket or jacket to stay warm and have him or her lie on his or her back with feet propped up to encourage blood flow to the brain. I can't stress enough, however, that 911 needs to be called and the bleeding needs to be stopped before anything else is done.

Quick Decisions

Is the blood spurting out? **YES** ▶ **CALL 911**

NO

Is the person...
pale?
sweaty?
dizzy?   **YES** ▶ **CALL 911**
confused?
stumbling?
drowsy?

AMPUTATIONS

Cutting off an arm, leg, or finger doesn't bleed nearly as much as you may think. Our bodies evolved to handle attacks by lions, tigers, and bears (oh my!), and we do a pretty good job of not bleeding to death when one of those predators decides to have part of us for a snack.

ON THE INTERNET

- firstaid.about.com/od/bleedingcontrol
- www.nlm.nih.gov/medlineplus/ency/article/000045.htm

III

Injuries and Illnesses

11

Help! I Don't Know Where to Start!

At the beginning of this book, I gave you six reasons to put the book down and call 911 immediately:

- Passing out
- Weakness on one side
- Won't waking up
- Bright red blood that won't stop squirting
- Sudden shortness of breath
- Someone isn't moving after getting hurt (punched, fell, struck by a car, etc.)

I'm assuming since you got this far that either you skipped the first chapter or you don't have those six problems. If you skipped the first chapter, then look at this list and see if your problem is there. If so, drop the book and pick up the phone; it's time to call 911.

Sometimes, if you aren't sure what kind of problem you're experiencing, it may be difficult to know where to start. Most things are covered in the table of contents. Got abdominal pain or back pain? Read Chapter 21. Feeling dizzy or faint? Read Chapter 22. Chest pain? Read Chapter 20.

Some medical complaints aren't specific to one easy explanation, or they just don't rate their own chapter. Either way, I've tried to cover those issues in this chapter. Look through these medical symptoms to find the right resource for you.

HEADACHE

If you have a sudden headache after hitting your head, turn to Chapter 14, "Knocking the Noggin." If your headache started suddenly without warning, there are a few things to consider:

- Confused, sweating, dizzy, or weak on one side, call 911 first. If you get bored while waiting for the ambulance to arrive, you can read Chapter 18, "Brain Matters."
- If you're in an extremely warm environment your headache might be a sign of dehydration. Read Chapters 22 and 24.
- Stuffy head, fever, or cough to go with your headache? Or do you have a stiff neck or a rash? Read Chapter 23.
- Anyone else in the house also complaining of a headache? Do you have a carbon monoxide alarm? Read about possible carbon monoxide poisoning in Chapter 27.

BLURRY VISION

Blurred or double vision can be a problem with the eyes or the brain. If you have a sudden loss of vision in one eye, especially if it looks as if you're staring down a tunnel, call 911. If you have sudden blurry vision in both eyes, read Chapter 18.

EARACHE

Feeling dizzy or nauseated? An earache could affect your balance. Any new earache is worth a call to the doctor.

SWOLLEN TONGUE/TROUBLE SWALLOWING

Sore throat with trouble swallowing could be a sign of an infection. Does it come with body aches or a fever? If so, read Chapter 23.

A swollen tongue can be a sign of an allergy or a medication reaction. If you have any trouble breathing or a choking sensation with your swollen tongue, call 911. While waiting for the ambulance, you can read Chapter 19.

WEAKNESS OR NUMBNESS

Weakness is one of the most common complaints in the over-65 crowd. Trying to figure it out can be very difficult. What is causing the weakness will only reveal itself by the other symptoms that come with the weakness:

- Do you have weakness only on one side? If so, call 911 immediately. The worst-case scenario is a possible stroke. Chapter 18 has more information on strokes.
- Weakness in both legs or in both arms at the same time is often caused by the same types of things as fainting. If you find yourself feeling like Superman just got a delivery of Kryptonite, turn to Chapter 22 for some possible causes.
- If your weakness comes during a heat wave or some other really hot time, look through Chapter 24 to see if heat exhaustion is the culprit. Definitely read Chapter 24 if you are cramping up.
- If your weakness comes with nausea and vomiting or diarrhea, you can try Chapters 22 or 23. If it's a fever, you see, Chapter 23 is the right place to be.
- Have diabetes? Eat a candy bar while reading Chapter 18.

NIGHT SWEATS OR COLD SWEATS

Busting out in a cold sweat, whether lying in bed in the middle of the night or sitting at the kitchen table in the middle of afternoon tea, could be a sign of a significant medical problem.

- Does the sweating come with chest pain or pressure in the chest? Call 911 (and read Chapter 20).
- Do you have cramping in the abdomen, constipation, diarrhea, nausea, or vomiting? Read Chapter 21.
- Feeling dizzy or weak? Read Chapter 22 or call 911.

NAUSEA AND VOMITING

It seems like almost everything makes us want to throw up: headaches, dizziness, brain injuries, food poisoning, paying taxes. . .

- Does anyone else in the house have nausea and vomiting? What about diarrhea for you or anyone else in the house? Read about food poisoning in Chapter 23.

- Fever? Also Chapter 23.
- Did you hit your head? Read about concussions in Chapter 14.

PAIN

Pain that happens without an obvious injury can be from all kinds of things. Pain is a sign from your body to your brain that something is wrong. It might be a little discomfort and it might be excruciating. This is one of those things that are completely personal. If you feel overwhelmed, either call the doctor or go to the emergency department.

- If the pain is in the chest, read Chapter 20.
- Arms or legs? Chapter 16.
- Belly? Chapter 21.
- Head? Go back to the first part of this chapter and read about headache. Or, read Chapters 14 and 18.

ON THE INTERNET

- www.mayoclinic.com/health/symptom-checker/DS00671
- firstaid.about.com/od/symptoms

12

Caring for Burns

Quick Decisions

Cool the burn with running tap water immediately

Charred or missing skin?
Burns on face or genitalia?
Burns encircling hands?
Burns encircling feet?
Blisters covering an area bigger than the belly?

YES to one or more

CALL 911

I f you've just been burned and you're reading this to find out what to do next, follow these steps:

- *Cool the burn with running water*: Put your burn under the faucet or the hose and just let the water cool your skin. It might take 20 minutes.
- If the skin is charred or missing, call 911.
- If the burn is on your face or genitals, call 911.
- If you can't read this book and cool the burn at the same time, then call 911.
- If you can read this book while you're cooling your burn, then read on.

TO CALL 911 OR NOT TO CALL 911?

How do you know when to call 911 and when to treat a burn at home? First let me just say that if you feel the burn is bad enough to call 911, go ahead and do that. In the worst cases, ambulances—or even helicopters—might take persons straight to a specialty burn center and skip the emergency room completely.

Figuring out if a burn is critical or just a minor thing can be a little complicated, which is why you should call if you think it's that bad. Paramedics use a combination of how much of the body is burned and how badly the burned skin is damaged to decide how critical a burn is.

If you're not sure and you're trying to decide whether to call 911 or not, look for burns with blisters. Burns with blisters that cover more than 10% of the body's surface (equal to about the size of the chest) are bad enough to call 911. Call 911 for any charred or missing skin, no matter how small the burn is.

We paramedics are not as worried about burns that just cause redness (like a mild sunburn), but if it covers enough of your body, it's probably still worth a trip—or at least a call—to the doctor.

Some burns are always bad no matter how small they seem to be. Always call 911 for these burns:

- *Face*: Burns cause swelling and breathing could become difficult if the burns are to the face.

FIRST-, SECOND-, OR THIRD-DEGREE?

Doctors, paramedics, and nurses classify burns as first-, second-, or third-degree. To us, how much the difference matters depends on which step of the treatment we're in. In the beginning—at the scene of the injury—paramedics only care whether a burn is first-degree or worse. Later, for severe burns that require surgery or long-term care, doctors and nurses need to know how deep burns are and care much more about the difference between second- and third-degree.

- *First-Degree Burns*: Superficial burns that only injure the top layer of skin are called first-degree burns. First-degree burns are red, tender, and tend to dry out. The top layer of skin will eventually peel off, but blisters don't form.
- *Second-Degree Burns*: Partial-thickness burns mean the top layer of skin is completely burned through and now the burn injury is down into the layer of the skin where hair grows and nerve endings live. Because those nerve endings are right there, second-degree burns hurt the worst. The second layer of skin is called the dermis, and it is filled with fluid. The fluid leaks out because of the injury and pushes the dead top layer (called the epidermis) up. As the top layer of skin separates and fills with fluid, it creates a blister. Second-degree burns can have small or very large blisters. In some cases, the top layer of skin just falls off and the raw skin underneath weeps fluid.
- *Third-Degree Burns:* Full-thickness burns mean the injury goes all the way through the top layer of skin and the second layer of skin. Third-degree burns are the worst type of burn. There is no such thing as a fourth-degree burn. Third-degree burns might not have any feeling because the nerve endings have been killed. However, any third-degree burns will be surrounded by extremely painful second-degree burns.

It's almost impossible to tell the difference between deep second-degree burns and third-degree burns outside of a hospital. Most health care workers can't tell the difference just by looking. If you suffer a burn that is severe and the skin is coming off, you should call 911 or go to the emergency room.

- *Hands or feet*: Burns that completely wrap around the hands or feet can swell up really badly and even lead to amputation if not treated soon. I'm not talking about a little blister on your finger from touching a hot oven. I'm talking about a bad burn that covers most of your hand or foot.
- *Genitals*: There's really nothing to say here. If you burn the nether regions you very much need to see a doctor immediately.

TREATING MINOR BURNS

Minor burns are those little blisters on your fingers from touching a hot pan or the sunburn you got from working in the backyard too long. Most of the time, you don't have to call 911 or even go to the doctor for those.

For the minor burns, do this:

1. *Stop the burning process*: Cool the minor burned area with cool running water for several minutes.
2. *Keep an eye out for blistering skin*: Blisters can form long after the burn happens, which is why it's so important to cool the burn completely. Blistering—or skin falling off—leaves the skin open to infection.
3. Burns with only red skin (no blisters) can be treated with a burn cream or first aid spray to reduce pain. Never put oil or butter on burns! Oil and butter might feel good going on, but they trap the heat and make the burn worse.
4. Cool water may also help with pain.
5. Ibuprofen (Advil, Motrin) or acetaminophen (Tylenol) can be used for pain of minor burns (redness, or just a little blister or two). For something stronger, you'll have to call your doctor.

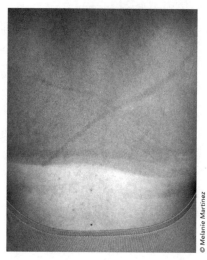
© Melanie Martinez

ON THE INTERNET

- www.nlm.nih.gov/medlineplus/ency/article/000030.htm
- firstaid.about.com/od/burninjuries

13

Have a Nice Trip;
See You Next Fall

Falls are associated with getting older and they have a certain stigma that doesn't come with other unforeseen medical emergencies. Based on talks with my older patients, falls come with much less warning than one might think there would be. Fall persons typically blame themselves, making the aftermath of a fall—especially a fall with significant injury—that much worse.

I promised at the beginning of this book not to preach. I figure you're old enough by now to decide how you want to live your life, and that includes choosing how to decorate your house, what you want to eat, and whether or not you plan to exercise. However, falls are the epitome of how an ounce of prevention really is worth a pound of cure.

According to the Centers for Disease Control and Prevention (CDC; falling is not a disease, but they still keep statistics on falls), one-third of all people 65 and over will fall each year. You're more likely to break something as a result of a fall than any other type of accident. Falls are also the most common cause of a brain injury in seniors—accounting for 46% of deadly outcomes.

I don't want to scare you—quite the opposite—I want to empower you. Indeed, the CDC says that once you fall, you might be afraid you'll fall again. You may start tiptoeing around and spending too much time on your butt instead of on your feet. Such a lack of activity will make you weak and unsure of yourself, increasing the chance that when you do get up and out (holidays with the grandkids, for example) you'll be more likely to take a tumble. No, I don't want you to be scared of being active; I want you to be confident and aware of what you need to do in order not to get hurt.

What does this have to do with decorating? Well, the most common causes of falls have to do with things around the house. Rugs go first: throw rugs and area rugs can bunch up or catch feet. It's worse if the rug has frilly edges or tassels.

Narrow walkways, especially between furniture, give you lots of things to trip over. Widen your path by getting rid of excess furniture and spreading things out.

Bathtubs are big culprits. Install handrails in the bathroom so you've got something to hold onto while entering and exiting the tub. Remember that the rails need to be installed correctly to support your weight; towel racks are not handrails (but properly installed handrails could certainly hold up a towel).

While we're calling the handyman to install handrails, it might not be a bad idea to update the lighting as well. Shedding a little more light on the room is a great way to reduce falls. If you can see where you're going, you're more likely to avoid tripping over things.

According to the CDC, women are twice as likely to break a hip from a fall as men. In fact, women are twice as likely to break anything as men are. Men, on the other hand, are 46% more likely to die from a fall than women.

Once we've done everything we can to make the house fall-proof, we should work on you. Falls seem pretty straightforward: you trip and you come crashing down. It's not really that simple.

Falls are from losing your balance. Balance is a complicated process that includes your brain taking in information about what position you're in (standing, sitting, or lying down), which direction you're moving, and what obstacles are in your way, then reacting to that information quickly enough to avoid the obstacles and keep you in control. To stay on top of all that information, we need to hear, see, and feel.

Some folks use walkers to help them stand and move about. It may seem like walkers are there to lean on, to prop you up. Instead, walkers and canes provide another point of contact for your brain to keep track of where you are. When you have your hand on a walker, a cane, or a railing, the touch is sending extra information to your brain so it can figure out exactly where you are, what position you are holding, and which direction you're facing.

Unfortunately, knowing where you are is only part of the battle. You need the strength and reflexes to react if something unexpected happens (like slipping on a newly waxed floor). Physical condition is an important part of getting older safely. Here's the preachy part: it's important to stay physically active because if you do not, you risk falling. Avoiding physical activity because you are afraid of falling means you won't have the strength and flexibility to stay vertical when things go wrong.

Here's what you need to do to avoid falling:

- Install grab bars, railings, and better lighting
- Get off your butt and get some regular exercise
- Don't be afraid to use tools like walkers and canes if you need them
- Throw out the throw rugs
- Get nonslip shoes

BEING ALONE

As a paramedic, I've treated dozens of folks who fell while home alone and had to lie on the floor for long periods of time. As it turns out, I met one of those people while writing this book.

Alice is a 78-year-old woman living alone with a nephew who comes to help her every day. One day her nephew arrived to find her lying on the floor. Alice had fallen late the night before and was unable to get to a phone. In fact, the phone was on the table just inches from Alice's fingertips, but she couldn't reach it.

Alice had a broken hip from her fall. Her hip was just too injured to allow her to reach up on the table. She told me on the way to the hospital that she'd recently talked to a medical alert company, but hadn't received the brochure yet.

Being alone is fine, but if you think you might have trouble getting up from a mishap, be sure to set up a plan for getting help.

Despite your best intentions and giving all those throw rugs to Goodwill, you still might take a tumble. If you're the one who falls, your most important concern is to get some help. When someone is home, you can yell for help, but what do you do if you're home alone?

If you think you might fall and you spend a lot of time alone, it's time to prepare for the worst. One option is to get one of those buttons to wear around your neck that you can push to call for help (see Chapter 2 on medical alert systems) or at least make sure there's a phone in each room (including bathrooms). When you can't stand up, you can at least work your way across a room if needed.

Instead of having a phone plugged into every wall of the house, you could get a cordless phone. There are two good reasons to carry your cordless phone when you're at home (not a cell phone; see Chapter 2 for the difference):

1. If you fall, you have a phone right there to call for help—family member or 911.
2. If the phone rings, you won't rush to answer it and trip over a piece of furniture on the way. Instead, you can simply pull it out of your pocket and say, "Hello?"

ON THE INTERNET

- www.stopfalls.org
- www.cdc.gov/features/fallrisks

14

Knocking the Noggin

Quick Decisions

Did the person get knocked out? **YES** → **CALL 911**

NO

Is the person...
dizzy?
confused?
stumbling?

Or have...
nausea?
vomiting?
headache?

YES → **CALL 911**

Taking one on the melon is a problem no matter how old you are. But if you'll recall, I mentioned in Chapter 13 how seniors get hurt more by falling than any other reason. We all relate breaking a hip with falls, but brain injuries are more common as we get older as well.

There are lots of structures you can damage when you knock your bean on the ground (or against the windshield, on a table, up against the wall, wherever you choose to hit your head). Your head is a lot of bone, a little muscle, some skin and other membranes, and, of course, a lot of brain. Plus, there's that beautiful face that Muhammad Ali was always so proud of. We don't want to mess up the face, right?

Since knocking your brain around isn't the same as putting an eye out, I'm going to separate the two issues. Chapter 17 has a section for impaled objects in the eye and Chapter 10 covers bloody noses. First, let's talk about the most important part: the brain.

TRAUMATIC BRAIN INJURIES

Whenever you smack your melon, paramedics worry about you injuring your brain. Hitting or shaking the brain can result in bleeding and swelling inside the skull, which is a problem because the skull is hard and sealed shut. A swollen or bleeding brain doesn't have anywhere to go; there's no place to let out the pressure.

The worst type of pressure comes from bleeding on the brain. Just like any other tissues or organs in the body, the brain can be cut, bruised, or ruptured. Sometimes, a weak artery in the brain—an aneurysm—will burst (this can happen with or without getting hit on the head). Whenever there's an injury causing bleeding or swelling on the brain, emergency treatment starts with getting to the emergency room (ER) immediately.

Blood thinners increase the chance for bleeding in the brain the same way they increase the chance for bruises or bleeding everywhere else. Anybody taking blood thinners who hits his or her head hard enough to get a goose egg should go to the emergency department to be checked out—especially if he or she is unconscious.

If someone hit his or her head—or was hit by something else—these are the signs that signal you to call 911:

- Is unconscious
- Short-term memory loss (person keeps repeating things or can't remember what he or she was doing)
- Unable to wake the person from sleeping (if you can't wake the person half an hour after going to sleep, call 911)
- Confusion
- Vomiting
- Dizziness
- Skull fracture

Besides trapping a swelling brain, that skull protects the brain from direct injury. It's our own built-in helmet. It's not a good idea to break it.

WHAT'S A CONCUSSION?

We hear a lot more about concussions in the news recently than we ever did before. When I started as a paramedic, concussions were considered no big deal. Indeed, the worst thing about a concussion was that it was hard to distinguish a "benign" concussion from a very dangerous bleed in the brain (at least without a CT scan).

Since those early days of ignorance, we've learned a lot more about concussions—enough to know that too many concussions can lead to a condition very similar to Parkinson's disease. We also know that we don't really know all that much.

Concussions come from getting hit on the head hard enough to cause the brain not to work right. Researchers haven't figured out exactly why the brain malfunctions, just that it does. It's kind of like when you drop your cell phone and it resets—nobody really understands why it does it, but it looks like it's still going to work.

So it used to be that if you got knocked out, but otherwise looked just fine, then no big deal. That's not the case anymore. Now we know if a hard bump on the head causes you to pass out, forget what happened, get confused, or throw up, we're calling 911.

Any bump on the head hard enough to crack the skull is hard enough to damage the soft brain underneath, so it's extremely important to call 911 if you think the skull is fractured. Here are some signs the skull could be broken:

- Soft or mushy to the touch (worst-case scenario)
- Bloody nose after a hit on the head
- Clear fluid draining from the ears or nose after a hit on the head
- Bruising behind the ear or around the eyes

What a Pain in the Neck

The most vulnerable part of our spine is the neck. It's not as protected and there's this little thing on top called the head that can get pulled, hit, twisted, and generally manipulated in ways that put the neck at risk for broken spine bones (vertebras) and damaged nerves (spinal cord injuries).

The worst-case scenario for a neck injury is permanent damage to the spinal cord that could lead to paralysis. Paramedics take neck injuries very seriously, but we don't want to make anyone uncomfortable by immobilizing the neck if we don't need to.

A good rule of thumb is that if the back of the neck hurts in the middle —right down the spine, especially to touch or movement—it's time to call 911.

On the Internet

- www.cdc.gov/concussion
- firstaid.about.com/od/concussions

15
Dressing Cuts and Scrapes

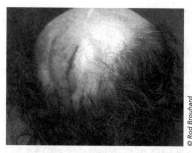
© Rod Brouhard

C uts and scrapes happen to everyone; you don't have to be a certain age. Indeed, I wouldn't be surprised if you spend more time doctoring the grandkids than doctoring yourself. Kids just have a way of finding things to cut themselves on.

Dressing or bandaging a wound depends on the type of wound. There are three main types of open wounds: lacerations, abrasions, and avulsions. Technically, amputations (cutting off an arm or leg) are also open wounds, but we covered those in Chapter 10.

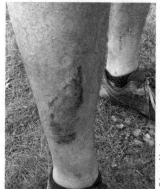
© Lynne Martinez

- *Lacerations* are accidental cuts (surgical cuts are called *incisions*) characterized by sometimes jagged edges that can be pushed together to close the cut.
- *Abrasions* are scratches that remove the top layer of skin and leave raw, sometimes bleeding skin behind.
- *Avulsions* are deeper than abrasions and look more like chunks of skin/tissue that have been removed. Sometimes avulsions are still hanging on by a flap, which means the avulsion can be closed.

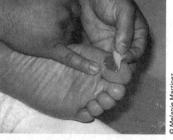
© Melanie Martinez

Before we get into how to properly dress a wound, the first thing to remember about any open wound is to control bleeding. Direct pressure with a piece of gauze or a clean cloth is the way to go. If the wound is on an arm or a leg, you can also elevate the limb above the level of your heart until bleeding stops (see Chapter 10 for more information on bleeding control).

87

Do I Need to See a Doctor?

There are several reasons to see a doctor for an open wound. Here are the definite times you should go to a doctor or the emergency department:

- Injured person has diabetes
- Animal or human bites (open wounds; it's not a big deal if it didn't break the skin)
- Can't get dirt or debris out of the wound
- Can't push the edges of the wound closed
- Numbness or decreased movement around an injury
- Uncontrolled bleeding; call 911 for this one

Besides these obvious injuries or having diabetes, you'll need to see a doctor if you haven't had a tetanus shot in the last 5 years and if you think you'll need stitches. Puncture wounds (holes in the skin from getting stuck or stabbed with something) should be evaluated by a doctor if you don't know how deep the hole is, especially if the puncture wound is in the chest, back, or belly.

HOW TO TELL IF YOU NEED STITCHES

Lacerations and some avulsions might benefit from stitches, but abrasions just have to heal. Whether a wound can be closed with stitches depends on several factors. Go to the doctor for stitches if any of these are present:

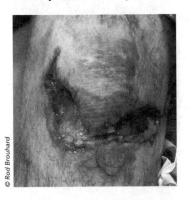

© Rod Brouhard

- Yellow, fatty tissue is visible in the cut
- Gaping wound where the edges can't be pushed together
- Injury is on the face or in a place where the skin stretches regularly (elbows, knees, hands, etc.)
- The injury is an avulsion with the chunk of skin still attached
- The injury happened less than 24 hours ago, although the longer you wait the less likely you will be able to get stitches

Very thin skin that's prone to tearing probably won't be able to handle stitches. If you have any doubts about whether you need stitches (or whether your skin can handle stitches), see a doctor.

CARE AND CLEANING OF YOUR WOUND

When bleeding has stopped, clean your open wound with water. Don't dress a wound without cleaning it first. Using a little soap around the edges is fine, but rinsing the wound with water is usually good enough for the raw, open parts. There's no need for those fancy antibacterial soaps. Rinse all the way, deep into the cut and rinse any soap away thoroughly.

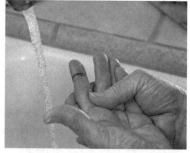

Tap water is perfectly fine for rinsing cuts; it's what all the big hospitals are using these days. There's nothing wrong with using sterile saline or sterile water, but it's not necessary at all. In fact, a plain bottle of water in a first aid kit can be used in case of a cut as well as to hydrate on a hot day.

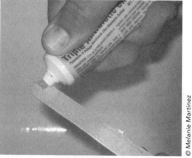

Once a wound is clean, keep it clean. If a cut or an abrasion gets dirty —even after it has been dressed— remove any dressing and clean it again. Keeping a wound clean is the best way to avoid infection.

Cleaning an open wound can make it bleed again. No problem, just use direct pressure to stop it. Usually, the bleeding will be minor. Once the bleeding stops, dress the wound.

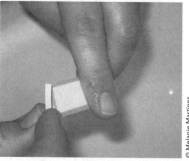

If you're going to use antiseptic ointment on the wound, put the ointment on a clean cotton swab or even a clean butter knife and dab it on. Don't squeeze it directly from the tube onto the open wound or you'll contaminate the whole tube. Antiseptic ointment is not always necessary and there are times you won't want to use it.

Cover the wound with an adhesive dressing. Don't put it on too tight. If an adhesive dressing won't stick because of body hair or if the skin is too delicate to handle adhesives, wrap the limb with a wide gauze roll.

Change dressings twice a day (about every 12 hours).

SHOULD I USE ANTISEPTIC OINTMENT?

Not if you're allergic to it—and you might not know that. Antiseptic ointment is a cream or gel usually containing three antibiotics: neomycin, bacitracin, and polymyxin. Antiseptic ointment is used to prevent infection and help healing.

Neomycin—one of the three antibiotics—causes a lot of allergic reactions.

Using antiseptic ointment helps some wounds heal quicker and with less pain. However, keeping the dressing fresh and moist is what makes the difference, rather than the infection-fighting properties of the antibiotics. An allergic reaction to antiseptic ointment can cause redness, itching, and burning—what doctors call *allergic contact dermatitis*—which looks a lot like an infected wound.

The problem is that after you get a cut, then clean it, cover it with ointment, and dress it, you expect it to get better. What happens when the wound and the surrounding skin get painful and red? If you think your wound is infected, you might put more ointment on it. Of course, that would make the dermatitis worse.

Sometimes you should simply trust your body to heal the way it's supposed to. If you have a problem that keeps you from healing like you should (diabetes or delicate skin, for example), talk to your doctor about how he or she wants you to handle cuts and scrapes.

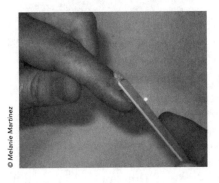
© Melanie Martinez

Lacerations that aren't going to get stitches should be held together with butterfly closures. Push the edges of the wound together and stick on the butterfly closures after the wound has been cleaned. Avulsions with a flap of skin can be closed the same way.

Once the wound is held together, you can dab on antiseptic ointment if you like (over the butterfly closures) and cover the wound as above. Superficial wounds that are not deep enough to see yellow fatty tissue do not need butterfly closures.

INFECTED WOUNDS

We all have nasty little bugs like streptococcus and staphylococcus running around on our skin just looking for ways to get in. When we get a cut or an abrasion (or a burn for that matter), we open the door to let these intruders attack. It's the reason we have to keep open wounds clean while they heal and change the dressings regularly. Look for these signs to tell if your open wound is getting infected:

- Tenderness or red skin (inflammation) around the wound
- Fever
- Swelling around the wound
- Numbness around the wound
- Red streaks around the wound

Tetanus is a very serious infection that can cause spasms in the jaw—called lockjaw—and even death. It's easily thwarted by a simple vaccine. If you haven't had at least three tetanus vaccinations and if the last one was more than 10 years ago, it's time to get another tetanus shot. Once you get a cut or a scrape, if your last tetanus shot is more than 5 years old, you should get another one.

WHAT ABOUT HYDROGEN PEROXIDE?

When I was growing up, my mom loved hydrogen peroxide and mercurochrome. As you may or may not have heard, mercurochrome is really dangerous and that's why you haven't seen it at the drug store lately.

Hydrogen peroxide on the other hand is readily available and you might be thinking that it's still okay to use on minor cuts and scrapes.

Nope.

Hydrogen peroxide is essentially water with an extra oxygen molecule in it. It bubbles a lot when it touches organic stuff like blood or raw skin. It does a great job of cleaning blood stains out of carpet and isn't too bad for canker sores. For cuts and scrapes, however, hydrogen peroxide not only doesn't help, it can even make things worse.

There are a few documented cases of hydrogen peroxide bubbles being absorbed into the bloodstream during surgical procedures and causing blockages. Hydrogen peroxide has also been shown to be very hard on skin, breaking it down and making it harder for the body to heal the wound. Leave the hydrogen peroxide in the cabinet and use water instead.

BLISTERS

Blisters are caused by burns, infections, or friction. Burns are covered in Chapter 12 and infections in Chapter 23. Blisters caused by friction can be pretty

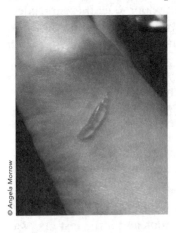

painful and are perfect spots for bacteria to grow. The same conditions that lead to blisters —warmth and moisture—are the conditions that bacteria love.

Deciding how to handle a blister depends on what you're doing at the time. If the blister is small, not too painful, and still intact (it still looks like a little bubble), then you can probably leave it alone. If it pops or if you're still doing whatever it is that caused the blister (walking or hiking, for example), then you'll want to treat it.

To treat a blister:

1. Clean it with a little soap and warm water. Pat it dry and put a little rubbing alcohol on the good skin around the blister.
2. Drain the blister with a needle. You'll have to clean the needle by holding it over a flame until the tip glows red, then let it cool without touching anything else. Carefully poke a little hole in the base of the blister with the needle. Don't remove the skin of the blister, you don't want a raw, tender spot. With a little pressure, help the blister ooze out all of the liquid inside.
3. Dress the blister with a little ointment and an adhesive bandage. You can use antiseptic ointment if you'd like or you can use a dab of petroleum jelly to keep it moist. Put the adhesive bandage on but don't make it too tight.
4. If you're going to still be walking, hiking, or doing whatever caused the blister in the first place, cut a piece of moleskin with a hole in the middle like a donut. Stick the moleskin to the skin around the blister to take pressure off the bubble. If you've drained the blister before putting the moleskin on, cover the whole thing with a bandage.

SKIN TEARS

Skin tears are cuts and scrapes of delicate skin that have a distinct look compared to wounds of healthier skin. Skin tears are just that: rips and tears of skin that has become very thin and usually very dry. Delicate skin that's susceptible to tearing is papery and sometimes feels kind of brittle.

Some folks are more susceptible to skin tears than others:

- Women more than men
- Lighter skin more than darker skin
- Those confined to a bed or wheelchair
- Bad diet (malnutrition)
- Taking corticosteroids for a long time
- Confusion or dementia
- Taking several medications
- Having lots of bruises
- Blood vessel, heart, lung, or vision problems
- Nerve pain or decreased sensation

Obviously, there are times when you're just more likely to hurt yourself: falling and bumping into things come to mind. If you're likely to get a bruise, and have healthy, strong skin, you're likely to get a skin tear when you have thin, delicate skin.

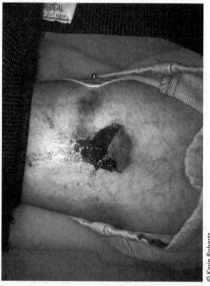

Managing skin tears is a little different from dressing cuts and scrapes on healthy skin. The same delicate skin that tore so easily the first time isn't going to do well with typical cleaning and dressing. You can't put a bandage on a skin tear because then you'll never be able to take it off. Even rinsing it with running water might make the tear bigger.

Despite how delicate skin tears are, the treatment is essentially the same: clean the wound with water or saline and cover it. How you cover it is the biggest change. Nonstick dressings are key. Dressings that come pre-moistened make good first aid bandages for skin tears.

To treat a skin tear:

1. Rinse the wound with running water or saline solution. Don't run the water too vigorously or you may end up doing more damage.

2. Let the skin tear dry completely or pat it dry very carefully.
3. Gently place the edges of the skin tear back together if possible. If part of the skin is missing, just do your best.
4. Cover the wound with a nonstick dressing. Common nonstick dressings are petroleum jelly gauze pads and transparent film dressings or absorbent acrylic dressings (Tegaderm). You can use Telfa-type pads as well, but I recommend the other options. Don't use plastic wrap: transparent film dressings look similar, but they allow oxygen through and promote healing.
5. Look for signs the skin tear is becoming infected: pain, redness, swelling, oozing, or odor. If it becomes infected, contact your doctor.
6. If you can't see the skin tear (if you used a dressing that's not transparent), you'll have to change the dressing every 2 or 3 days. When taking off a dressing from a skin tear, always peel it off in the same direction as the tear, not backward, or you risk opening the tear back up again.
7. If you did use a transparent dressing, keep an eye on the skin tear daily until it heals. If the dressing gets contaminated or damaged, peel it off, rinse the wound, and replace the dressing.

Skin tears are more complicated than I'm giving them credit for here, so if you have questions about your skin type, ask your doctor for advice. Sometimes the old saying about "an ounce of prevention" is the best way to handle skin tears—don't get them.

There are some activities that are heavily associated with skin tears in folks with thin skin:

• Using walkers and canes
• Putting on and taking off stockings or socks
• Removing medical tape
• Moving back and forth between bed and wheelchair

If you are prone to skin tears, wearing long sleeves can help. The best thing you can do is keep your skin healthy and moisturized. Eat well, stay active, and use lotion to avoid dry skin.

PRESSURE SORES

Pressure sores (or pressure ulcers) are areas of damaged skin from staying in contact with another surface too long and not moving. Pressure sores are common in folks who are confined to bed and don't move much.

Treating pressure sores at home can be difficult. Usually, treatment requires an evaluation by a health care provider to determine how bad the pressure ulcer is and to develop a plan for treatment. The most important thing you can do at home is to learn how to recognize pressure sores and know when it's important to start looking for them.

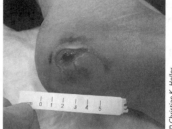

First of all, pressure sores are most likely to show up when:

- The person is bedbound and cannot get up
- The person is paralyzed
- The person is frequently incontinent (even if he or she wears an adult diaper)
- The person has thin skin (the kind susceptible to skin tears)

Pressure sores start off looking red and irritated and progress to a soft, and often very tender, ulcer. Please pardon the crude example, but pressure sores feel very similar to a piece of rotting fruit. These can be very dangerous to the patient and may lead to life-threatening infections. If you think you see a pressure sore, call the doctor.

Bruises

Bruises happen to everyone, but as we get older they happen more frequently. Delicate skin and blood thinners are two culprits, but all of us bruise more easily with age.

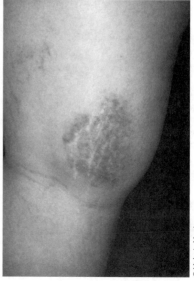

For the most part, bruises are harmless. If they appear in an area where bruises are likely (shins, arms, thighs, etc.), then the only concern is cosmetic and whether the bruise is causing any pain.

Treat a simple bruise with ice and elevation. Remember, only put ice on for 15 to 20 minutes and leave it off for at least the same amount of time. Make sure there's something like a dry towel or cloth between the ice pack and your skin or you risk frostbite. If you can, elevate the injured arm or leg above the level of your heart to minimize the bruising.

After a few days, you can switch to heat instead of ice if you want. Theoretically, heat promotes healing of the bruise.

Bruising on the face, chest, back, or abdomen that doesn't come from a fall or getting hit needs to be evaluated by a doctor. This is especially important if the bruise comes with pain.

On the Internet

- www.nlm.nih.gov/medlineplus/bruises.html
- firstaid.about.com/od/softtissueinjuries

16
Breaks and Sprains

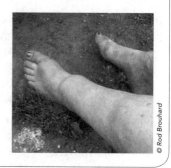

© Rod Brouhard

Broken bones are more common as we age. Calcium, the mineral most responsible for keeping bones hard, is lost from bone tissue. As calcium is lost, bones get more brittle and break more easily.

When major amounts of calcium are lost, miniscule spaces develop in the bone tissue where the calcium used to be. It's called *osteoporosis*. Women are more prone to osteoporosis than men are, but regardless of whether you have a diagnosis of osteoporosis—or whether you're male or female—your bones aren't going to be as strong now as they were 20 years ago.

There are other injuries that can put us on the sidelines for almost as long as broken bones. Sprains and strains are injuries of the muscles, tendons, and ligaments we use to move our bodies around. Ligaments hold the joints together while muscles and tendons move them. Tearing or stretching any of these can be nearly as painful and debilitating as a fracture.

The symptoms of strains, sprains, and broken bones are pretty similar. We're going to treat them essentially the same way regardless of what it looks like on the X-ray, despite the fact that most health care providers (and patients) tend to consider a broken bone worse than the other possibilities. The most common symptoms in all cases are:

- Pain
- Swelling
- Bruising
- Inability to move
- Inability to bear weight on the joint or limb

It isn't necessary to have all these symptoms for the injury to be a sprain or a broken bone. Likewise, just because you have all these symptoms doesn't mean you've broken a bone.

Most of the time, it's not necessary to call 911. You should call 911 for an injury if you can't get to a doctor any other way, or if it makes you immobile. In many cases, you can treat a sprain or a strain at home. Broken hips and broken ribs are covered specifically later in this chapter.

Visit a doctor if you think you have a sprain if the part of your body you've sprained:

- Has severe pain (more than you can handle)
- You can't put any weight on it
- Looks different from the uninjured joint (swelling doesn't count)
- You can't move it
- You can't walk more than four steps on it
- There is numbness in any part of it
- Redness or red streaks spread out from the injury
- Has been sprained several times before
- There is pain, swelling, or redness over a bony part of your foot, rather than the ankle

R.I.C.E.

Whether you go to a doctor or not, you should treat any injury with R.I.C.E. (rest, ice, compression, elevation)

R.I.C.E. helps cut down on inflammation and swelling. Using these four techniques slows blood flow to an injury, so R.I.C.E. should only be used as an early treatment to cut back on swelling. Tomorrow or the next day you'll want to increase blood flow to help healing.

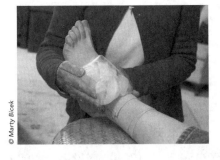
© Marty Bicek

- *Rest.* Take a load off, literally. Stay off your injured leg or avoid using your messed up arm. Whatever you did, give it a rest for the next couple of days.
- *Ice.* Ice the injury to help keep the pain and swelling down. Don't put the ice pack right on the skin and definitely be careful how long you leave it on there. Be especially careful if you have poor circulation. My daughter got frostbite from an ice pack when she was a healthy teenager. It's not hard to do. Every couple of hours, put ice on the injury for 10 minutes, take it off for 10 minutes, and put it back on for 10 more, then take a break from the ice. Studies show that this process helps cut back on pain for ankle injuries (and common sense says it will help for other injuries as well).

- *Compression.* Wrap an elastic bandage (Ace bandages are the most common) around the injury. Don't wrap it too tight, but not too loosely either. You should easily be able to slip two fingers under the wrap.
- *Elevation.* Prop up your injured arm or leg higher than your heart. It's easier to do this for an injured leg if you lie down and rest.

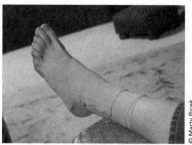

So, to sum up: Rest on the couch with your ankle wrapped in an elastic bandage and propped up on a pillow while putting ice on it for 10 minutes at a time twice every couple of hours. Simple, no?

If you're not feeling better after a couple days of using R.I.C.E., then you need to call the doctor. If you do start feeling better, let it heal and stop icing and elevating.

If you aggravate your injury while it's healing, you can use R.I.C.E. again, but don't overdo it. Like many things, R.I.C.E. is good in moderation.

DISLOCATIONS

There's one more type of joint injury that's usually considered as bad as— and sometimes worse than—a fracture: a dislocation. A dislocation happens when a joint comes apart. A joint is a place in the body where two or more bones come together, like an elbow, knee, or hip.

A joint dislocation is a big deal. When a bone gets pulled out of alignment with the other bones in a joint, the joint no longer works correctly. It can't move the way it's supposed to and it is probably the most painful type of injury covered in this chapter.

Joint dislocations need to be treated in the emergency department. If you dislocate a shoulder, a finger, a toe, or an elbow and want to go to the ER by car, only go if someone else can drive you. If you dislocate a knee (not the kneecap, see following) or a hip, call 911.

One thing to note: it's a much bigger deal to dislocate an elbow or a knee than anything else. Knees and elbows have strong ligaments and tendons to hold them in place and pulling all that apart is serious business. The tendons and ligaments in hips and shoulders are more spread out and aren't as strong. It takes much less energy to dislocate a shoulder than it does to tear apart the elbow.

Kneecaps (officially called the *patella*) are one of the most common bones to dislocate and one of the easiest to fix. You can tell a kneecap is dislocated because it will slide to the side (usually the outside) instead of being right in the middle where it belongs. In most cases, you can slip the kneecap back into place while straightening the knee—just be sure to do both at exactly the same time.

The longer you leave a kneecap out of place, the more damage is done to the tissues around it.

Hip Fractures

We all begin to worry just a little bit more about breaking a hip as we get older. The hip joint is where the femur (giant thigh bone) meets the pelvis. The top of the femur has a ball on the end of it that fits into a socket in the pelvis.

Broken hips usually happen because the head of the femur (the *ball* part of the *ball and socket* hip joint) snaps off at the *neck*, a narrow part of the femur just below the head. Often, hip fractures aren't really fractures at all but hip dislocations instead. Sometimes it's possible to tell the difference based on how the injured leg looks, but most of the time you'll need an X-ray.

The most common cause of a broken hip is falling. In order to avoid broken hips, you should avoid falling (see Chapter 13).

There are some common signs and symptoms of broken hips, but you need not have them all for a hip to be fractured.

• It hurts. In many cases, this will be the only symptom.
• Can't move the hip.
• The injured leg is shorter than the uninjured leg.
• The injured leg is rotated in or out.

If you have a history of osteoporosis, it's possible to have what's known as a spontaneous hip fracture (breaks without hitting it or falling). Those are pretty rare, however, and if your bones are that brittle you should already know it's a possibility.

There's nothing you can do for a broken hip at home. If you or some-one in the house takes a tumble and can't move the hip—or it hurts too much when tried—call 911. Here are some things to do until the ambulance gets there:

• Make yourself or the other person as comfortable as possible until the ambulance arrives
• Follow any instructions the 911 operator gives you
• Don't have anything to eat or drink

Hip fractures definitely get more common as we age because it doesn't take as much force to break brittle bones as it does to break healthy ones. Because of that, the younger you are when you break a hip, the more dangerous it is. No matter how old the person is, if you suspect a broken hip, call 911.

BROKEN RIBS

Like hips, the older and more brittle your ribs are, the easier it is to break them. Rib fractures are important not because there's anything we can do for them. There's not. But because of where they are. Your ribs are there to protect your heart and lungs. A rib fracture can puncture a lung or pierce the heart. A bunch of broken ribs (rare even in the elderly) can make it very hard to breathe, even when the lungs are intact.

Most broken ribs come from car accidents. If your bones are pretty brittle, you can break a rib with forceful coughing like you might get with pneumonia (see Chapters 19 and 23). Ribs can also break from the usual suspects: trips and falls.

Ribs don't usually snap in half. They crack and hurt like the dickens. If they do snap, they can start puncturing lungs and the heart like I mentioned before. A punctured lung can collapse (called a *pneumothorax*, see Chapter 19), making it very hard to breathe.

Once in a while, a section of ribs breaks away from the rest of the rib cage. The muscles are still there to hold everything in place, but with the ribs shattered like that the area becomes soft. When that happens, the section of broken ribs "floats" in and out when you try to breathe, a very painful emergency condition called *flail chest*.

The best way to tell if a rib is broken is by pain. If you got smacked in the chest with a steering wheel, floor, baseball bat, or a horse kicked you and it now hurts to breathe, it's worth getting checked out at the emergency department for possible rib fractures. If you've been coughing a lot and now you can't take a deep breath or cough because it hurts too much, it's also time to head for the ER.

Some other telltale signs:

- Ribs are very tender to touch
- You feel a "crunchy" feeling under the skin—it's called *crepitus* and it comes from broken bone bits rubbing together
- A section of your rib cage moves in the opposite direction of the rest of your chest when you breathe—a sign of *flail chest*
- Severe shortness of breath
- Coughing blood
- Blood in the urine

THE DIFFERENCE BETWEEN A FRACTURE AND A BREAK

Let's clear this right up: a fracture is a break and a break is a fracture. They are one and the same.

My son broke his leg in football practice. He was kind of a little guy his freshman year and a big kid landed on his leg in tackle drills.

His mom and I picked him up from school and spent the next whole day at his doctor's office, the imaging center, and the orthopedic surgeon's office. When my son returned to school 2 days later, everyone wanted to know if he had a fracture or a break.

A fracture, he was told, is just a crack. But a break meant it was busted into smithereens. Even his coaches thought this way.

My son educated them all—coaches as well—that indeed a fracture is just another name for a break. His coaches didn't believe him. I had to write a blog about it so he could send his coaches there to read it for themselves.

So to clear up any confusion, let me be crystal clear: a fracture and a break are the exact same thing. It's like calling fuchsia pink or pink fuchsia. Really, who cares?

Let's face it, if you got hit in the chest hard enough that you think you may have broken a rib, you should go to the ER. Broken ribs—especially more than one—can make it hard to breathe and can lead to pneumonia or other complications.

If all you have is a simple, single rib fracture, the doctor will probably just give you some pain medication and let it heal. We don't do anything for broken ribs anymore (no wrapping or splinting). If it's worse than that, your doctor may need to admit you to the hospital and provide oxygen or other emergency treatment.

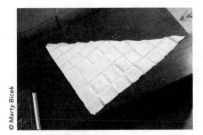

© Marty Bicek

BROKEN COLLARBONES AND DISLOCATED SHOULDERS

Because of how close they are to each other and the way they feel, broken collarbones (fractured clavicles) and dislocated shoulders are treated pretty much the same. These are not life-threatening emergencies but they sure do hurt and both of them are worthy of the emergency department, if not 911. If you decide to take yourself to the hospital, you can stabilize an injured collarbone fairly easily.

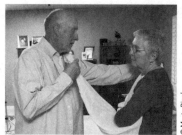

The most important thing to remember with shoulder and collarbone injuries is to support the injured arm with a sling of some sort. Slings can be made with a triangular bandage if you have one in your first aid kit or you can be clever with a button-up shirt or jacket. To use a triangular bandage:

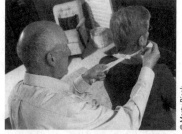

1. Unfold the triangular bandage completely. One side will be longer than the other two.
2. Put the middle of the long side of the triangular bandage under the hand/wrist. Slip one corner behind the arm up to the neck and the other corner in front of the arm to the neck.
3. Tie the corners behind the neck.
4. Tie a knot in the corner at the elbow to provide a little support. This keeps the arm from slipping out of the sling.

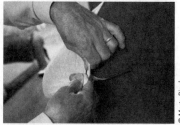

If you don't have a triangular bandage, a little ingenuity can still get the job done. A button-up shirt can be used to make a sling by folding the shirt tail up and over the injured arm. Either pin or button the tail in place.

Once the arm is supported with a sling, ice the shoulder just like you would with R.I.C.E. Unlike an injured leg or arm, you're not going to elevate or wrap an elastic bandage around the injury. Head for the hospital but don't drive yourself. Have someone else take you.

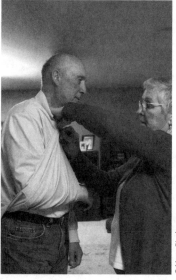

Broken Humerus (It's Not Funny)

The upper arm bone from the shoulder to the elbow is called the *humerus*. It's the thickest, hardest bone in the arm. You can be sure, a humerus fracture is no laughing matter (sorry, I couldn't resist). Like the collarbone and a shoulder dislocation, the humerus doesn't necessarily require 911, but it does need to be treated in the emergency department.

Splinting a humerus fracture is a lot like slinging a shoulder injury, but you're going to do one extra step. After you've fashioned a sling out of a triangular bandage, a jacket, or a shirt, you should wrap a wide bandage around the chest and the arm just to provide a little more stability.

Anytime you put a splint or a sling on an injury, you want to make sure the person can still feel and wiggle his or her fingers. Plus, you want to compare the hand on the injured arm to the hand on the uninjured arm, to make sure they're the same temperature and color. If the hand on the injured arm gets cold, pale, blue, numb, or can't move, call 911.

Once you've got a sling and a wrap (called a swath) on the person's injured arm, you can go to the hospital. If you're the person with the break, you need a driver. If it hurts too much to ride in the car—or you're by yourself—call 911.

Broken Wrist

If you fall and don't catch yourself, you might end up with a broken hip like we discussed earlier. If you put your hand out to catch yourself, you could end up with a broken wrist. I know; it's like you're darned if you do and darned if you don't.

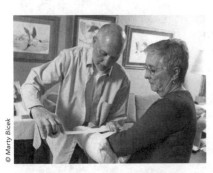

A broken wrist is often called a spoon fracture because of the way it usually looks. They're very common in kids but they can happen to adults of all ages as well.

The most important thing to do for a wrist fracture is to support it. One easy way to do that is to wrap a pillow around the arm. Make sure you support the hand as well as the arm and don't bend the wrist. A good trick is to put something in the hand to hold onto while you splint the wrist—use an empty toilet paper tube or a rolled up sock.

Once the splint is in place, ice the wrist, elevate it, and take it to the hospital because you need an X-ray and a doctor.

KEEP YOUR HANDS AND FEET INSIDE THE RIDE AT ALL TIMES

Broken hands, broken feet, broken fingers, and broken toes usually all show up as painful, bruised, and swollen. None of these injuries needs 911 unless there's no other way to get treatment. In most cases, treat with R.I.C.E. and call your doctor.

If you think a toe or a finger is dislocated, you can go to the emergency department to get it *reduced*, fancy medical terminology for "put back into place." On your way to the hospital, be sure to elevate and ice it if possible.

ON THE INTERNET

- firstaid.about.com/od/breaksandsprains
- www.aaos.org

17
Slings and Arrows

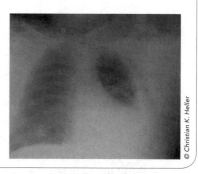

© Christian K. Heller

Puncture wounds don't look much different from other types of lacerations, except that you can't tell how deep they go. The basic definition of a puncture wound is that it's deeper than it is wide. Puncture wounds are common in car accidents and falls (landing on something sharp), or in drive-by shootings and knife fights (if you have a lot of those, this might be the wrong book for you).

The danger of a puncture wound is that unless you know exactly what caused the wound and how it happened, you can't be sure how deep it is or what anatomy is damaged under the surface. There is likely to be at least some bleeding under there, even if you can't see it oozing out of the hole.

Taking care of puncture wounds is about controlling whatever bleeding you can and protecting the wound from getting infected as much as possible.

Controlling bleeding is done as it is for any other type of cut: direct pressure and elevation. Use gauze pads to encourage clotting and don't forget to keep pressure on there for at least 10 minutes. Tourniquets are rarely necessary and take special training to use correctly.

Deciding when to call 911 for a puncture wound is based on where the wound is and how deep it is. Punctures of unknown depth to the neck, chest, abdomen, back, pelvis, or thigh should get a 911 call. Punctures that won't stop bleeding should also get a 911 call.

A hole in the chest can lead to a collapsed lung. Keep an eye on anyone with a puncture wound to the chest or the back for trouble breathing. Remember, if they have a puncture to the chest or back, you should have called 911. Watch for trouble breathing while you're waiting for the ambulance to arrive.

After you stop any bleeding, you can clean the wound just like you would any other type of cut. Punctures might need stitches as well.

COLLAPSED LUNG

You've probably heard of a collapsed lung before. The first time I heard the term I thought of a balloon with all the air leaking out of it, kind of wrinkly and loose. Because lungs don't actually work like balloons, they don't collapse like them either. Something has to push a lung down—usually air or blood collecting between the lung and the wall of the chest.

When you get a puncture wound in the chest, it can allow air to suck in through the hole when you breathe. It's even called a *sucking chest wound*. To stop that from happening, we seal chest wounds with airtight dressings. While waiting for an ambulance, you could do the same thing with your hand. Just cover the wound and don't let any air through.

When the paramedics get there, they'll seal it up for you.

Small punctures that don't need stitches and aren't on an area that requires you to call 911 can just get cleaned, dabbed with antiseptic ointment if you so desire, and covered with a bandage. Change the bandage every day until it's healed. If the puncture looks like it's getting infected (swelling, redness, or oozing pus), call your doctor.

If your puncture wound comes from a dog, cat, or other animal bite, you should go to the doctor to have it cleaned. There's a lot of potential for infection from bites—even human bites. Plus, you'll need to evaluate the possibility of rabies from some animals (the most common rabies infections come from bats and raccoons).

You can use acetaminophen (Tylenol) or ibuprofen (Motrin or Advil) to relieve the pain of a minor puncture. For the bigger wounds that need a doctor's help, ask the doctor what to take for pain.

Sometimes, whatever made the puncture wound is still there. When it's a big thing that made a big puncture and it's still there, we call it an impaled object. When it's a small thing that made a small hole and it's still there, we call it a splinter.

SPLINTER REMOVAL

There isn't an official size difference between that which is a splinter and that which is too big to be considered a splinter. Essentially, if it's superficial (it doesn't go deeper than the fatty tissue below the skin), it's a splinter.

Deeper than that and you might consider it an impaled object—unless it doesn't look *too* big—in other words, use your own judgment.

You can remove splinters at home. First, make sure the wound is not infected. Some splinters are more likely to get infected than others. The type of material makes the difference. If the splinter is organic—bone or wood—it has a better chance of becoming infected. Look for these signs of infection:

- Redness
- Swelling
- Pus draining from the wound
- Severe pain even without movement

Assuming it's not infected, you can remove a splinter by doing the following:

1. Wash your hands thoroughly before taking out a splinter. Wash with soap and water for at least 30 seconds.
2. Before attempting to grab the splinter with tools, try to squeeze it out like popping a zit. See if you can work it out of the skin. If you get it out far enough, grab it with a pair of tweezers.
3. If you can't squeeze it out, clean a sewing needle with povidone-iodine solution. Don't use rubbing alcohol or alcohol prep pads unless that's absolutely all you have available. Povidone-iodine solution is the best bet.
4. Wash the splinter wound and surrounding skin with soap and warm water. Putting povidone-iodine solution directly on the wound will also help.
5. Use the needle to separate the skin over the splinter just enough to grab the splinter with tweezers. Pull it straight out.
6. If a needle doesn't work, you can use a pair of nail clippers to remove the skin—be sure to also clean the nail clippers with povidone-iodine solution.
7. Finally, wash the wound one more time with warm water and soap. Don't be afraid to use more povidone-iodine solution.

Splinters don't usually hurt bad enough to take medication. If the area gets very tender, you can try a bee sting swab to numb it.

Splinters under a fingernail are called *subungual splinters.* They might be a bigger problem. If you can reach the tip of a subungual splinter with a pair of tweezers, you may be able to pull it out.

If you can't pull a subungual splinter out by tweezers you have two options: go to the doctor or wait for nature to run its course. If you go to the doctor, he might be able to snip away enough fingernail to reach the splinter. If you wait, natural fingernail growth should eventually push the splinter out. However, you may have to wait several days. If you choose to wait, watch the area closely for signs of infection.

Any time you get a splinter, you want to make sure you're up to date on your tetanus shot. If it's been more than 5 years since your last tetanus vaccination, go let the doctor pull out your splinter and get a tetanus booster.

Regardless of where the splinter is, natural skin growth should eventually push it out. There's no hurry, so if you have to wait until you can be clean and sanitary, that's fine. Don't take splinters out on a camping trip or other dirty area.[4]

IMPALED OBJECT

If it's bigger than a splinter (you decide how big that is), then it's an impaled object. The basic rule for impaled objects is if it went in, leave it in.

Impaled objects plug the hole they create. Therefore, by leaving an impaled object in place, you keep the area from bleeding. It's a little like leaving the cork in the bottle.

You also don't want an impaled object to wiggle too much while it's stuck in the body. The more it wiggles, the more damage it does. If you are dealing with an impaled object, call 911. Paramedics will secure the object in place, shorten it if possible, and take you to the hospital.

At the hospital, doctors will decide if the impaled object will have to be removed surgically. I've seen people impaled with crochet hooks, toothbrushes, and broomsticks, all needing surgery to remove.

IMPALED OBJECT IN THE EYE

Like Mom says: it's all fun and games until somebody pokes an eye out.

Impaled objects in the eye have shown up in first aid books since first aid books were invented. I think it's because somebody came up with the paper cup idea for a pencil in the eye and authors love to include clever ideas in first aid books.

Here's what you need to know about impaled objects in the eye: cover both eyes so there's no desire to look around (remember, we don't want impaled objects to wiggle) and call 911. The paramedics will know what to do with your eye emergency.

RIDING THE BROOMSTICK

The truck driver had a routine. After he delivered the feed to the dairy, he swept out the trailer to make sure the customer got the entire delivery. When he was done sweeping out the "walking floor" trailer, he tossed the broom and jumped down behind it.

That's when we got called.

The broom handle bounced on the concrete and was sticking straight up by the time the driver was jumping out. The broom handle pierced him right through the groin and went all the way to his collarbone. He was hurting for sure, but doing pretty well. True to form, despite how severe the impaled object was, there wasn't a drop of blood.

When we emergency folks got there, we secured the impaled broom handle, took the bristle head off and sent him to the hospital in a helicopter. Surgeons were able to remove the broomstick and our driver has a terrible scar, but didn't lose a single organ from his ordeal.

Today, the broom handle decorates a corner of my office at home.

ON THE INTERNET

- www.nlm.nih.gov/medlineplus/ency/article/000043.htm

18

Brain Matters: Confusion and More

There are lots of things that can affect the brain. Some of the material that is covered in this chapter doesn't seem to have much in common with the brain, but as we'll see, when the problem gets to the brain you'll notice it.

Your brain is picky. It likes to be warm, but not too warm; sweet, but not too sweet; and to be under pressure, but not too much pressure. To do all this, the brain needs blood to carry oxygen and sugar. When your brain doesn't like what it's getting (or not getting), it acts out, malfunctions, or just plain shuts down.

It's always a good idea to call 911 whenever the brain is malfunctioning. Look for these signs to call 911:

- Sudden confusion
- Sudden slurred speech
- Weakness or numbness on one side or *facial droop*
- Inability to speak or speaking gibberish
- Sudden trouble walking or sudden dizziness
- Sudden severe headache, especially if the person has never had bad headaches before
- Sudden trouble seeing or blurred vision in one or both eyes
- Seizures (read further for more information on seizures)

All of these things can be symptoms of a stroke, but they can also be caused by other conditions such as low blood sugar, seizures, infection, or certain kinds of poisoning, all of which I'll cover later. For now, let's just talk about stroke.

When I was a brand new paramedic, I was taught that nothing could be done for a stroke (sometimes called a *brain attack* and known among health care providers as a *cerebrovascular accident*). Once the brain was injured, we were told, the damage was permanent.

Since then, lots of work has been done and health care providers have many more tools in their toolbox for treating stroke. All of the tools are in the hospital, however, so if you ever suspect a stroke, call 911 immediately.

STROKES

A stroke is a medical condition of the brain. It occurs when a portion of the brain is suddenly starved for oxygen.

There are two very different causes of stroke:

- Ischemic stroke is a blockage of a blood vessel in the brain that stops blood flow to a section of brain tissue. This is the more common type of stroke and usually the blockage comes from a blood clot.
- Hemorrhagic stroke occurs when a blood vessel in the brain bursts and causes bleeding in or around the brain.

WHY IS IT "STROKE" AND WHAT THE HECK IS A MINI-STROKE, ANYWAY?

The name *stroke* comes from an ancient belief that folks suffered this terrible and sudden fate at the "stroke of God's hand." The term has stuck, despite an attempt by some in the medical field to change it to a "brain attack." The official medical term for stroke is *cerebrovascular accident (CVA)*.

Sometimes, the symptoms of a stroke will come and go all by themselves without any medical treatment. It may happen within seconds or it could take a day. Often, doctors will say the person suffered a *mini-stroke*. In the medical field, we call it a *transient ischemic attack (TIA)*.

As we learn more about the brain and conditions that affect the brain, we are beginning to understand there's more than one kind of transient episode that might cause symptoms similar to strokes.

On February 13, 2010, a television reporter covering the Grammy Awards had sudden trouble speaking live on the air. The reporter, Serene Branson, shared with the world after that night that she'd suffered a migraine headache and the symptoms were from the migraine. In years past, that would most certainly have been categorized as a mini-stroke.

Ischemic stroke can be treated with medications that dissolve the clot, but there's only a small window of time for the medication to be given. It's really important to call 911 right away if you think you or someone else might be having a stroke. The person will have to be transported to the hospital and a CT scan of the brain is necessary to tell if it's ischemic or hemorrhagic before any medication can be given.

DIABETES AND LOW BLOOD SUGAR

The most common emergency for diabetics is *hypoglycemia* (low blood sugar). It might seem backwards, since diabetes is a condition of too much sugar, but the treatment for diabetes makes it hard to control blood sugar without going too low.

When the blood sugar gets low, either from taking too much medication or taking the right amount of medication and eating too little, the brain starves for sugar and begins to malfunction. As the brain malfunctions, several things can happen:

- Confusion
- Fumbling fingers
- Shaking or trembling (diabetics call this "the shakes")
- Slurred speech
- Trouble walking
- Sweating
- Passing out

Fixing low blood sugar can be as simple as giving the person some sugar or other simple carbohydrates. The easiest form of sugar to give is usually juice. Just have the person drink a glass of orange or apple juice, as long as he or she can follow commands. Don't try to give the person juice or food if he or she can't swallow it.

If the person is unconscious, it's time to call 911. Paramedics will respond and they can give sugar intravenously. The person may not even need to go to the hospital after getting sugar, but that will depend on the rules governing paramedics in your area.

After getting the blood sugar level up with something sugary, you'll want the patient to eat something with protein to help the blood sugar stabilize. When I respond by ambulance to diabetic patients with low blood sugar, my favorite meals to feed them (after giving the sugar) are peanut butter sandwiches or fried eggs.

I have to admit, it looks pretty funny to be having an egg fried in your kitchen by a paramedic, but we make a really mean breakfast.

Anytime you or a loved one has an episode of low blood sugar, you need to contact the doctor to let him or her know what happened. If you're suffering low blood sugar often, it may be time to adjust your medication. Your doctor will need to know about any visits from the ambulance crew or trips to the emergency department in order for him or her to make the right decisions for your health.

Seizures

Seizures are scary to watch, probably even more than they are scary to have. As dramatic as a seizure can be, it's important to understand that seizures are more of a symptom than a problem. Seizures tell us that something is wrong with the brain. Sometimes, health care providers might even be able to tell which part of the brain is affected by the way a seizure looks.

There are a few different types of seizure, but these are the most common:

- *Petit mal:* These seizures can look like somebody just gazing off into the distance, almost trance-like. In some cases, petit mal seizures might have a little minor twitching or facial tics. Most of the time, the person looks catatonic.
- *Grand mal:* The big, full-body convulsions that everyone thinks of when we talk about seizures. Grand mal seizures are also called tonic-clonic seizures.
- *Focal seizures:* When only a part of the body is involved in a seizure, or suffers seizure-like activity, we call that a focal seizure, partial seizure, or focal motor seizure. Simple focal seizures do not affect awareness whereas complex focal seizures cause a loss of alertness or consciousness.

Seizures generally come in three phases, especially grand mal seizures:

- *Aura (also known as pre-ictal):* The aura is the first part of the seizure. Some persons can feel or otherwise recognize an aura and prepare for the oncoming seizure activity, but many persons don't even know they're having it. In either case, the aura is the beginning of the entire seizure process. By the time the person is feeling an aura, the seizure is starting to happen. Auras can be very quick or last several minutes.
- *Ictal phase:* The seizure itself (jerking motions and muscle contractions) is called the ictal phase. The ictal phase can last anywhere from a few seconds to more than an hour.

- *Postictal phase:* After the shaking stops there is a recovery period known as the postictal phase. During this time the person will be groggy and confused, gradually returning to normal.

Seizures are rarely life-threatening and usually don't require much treatment. Because seizures are symptoms of other problems, determining the cause of the seizure becomes very important for health care providers. Patients with chronic seizure disorders like epilepsy are usually controlled by taking prescription medication and their doctors won't be very worried by the occasional seizure.

For people who don't normally suffer from seizures, having one means something in the body has changed and has affected the brain. There are some very common causes of seizures in people who don't normally have them:

- Fever, especially in children
- Sudden loss of consciousness (passing out)
- Low blood sugar
- Injury to the brain
- Infection or parasites in the brain
- Stroke

With all these possible causes of seizures, it can feel overwhelming as you wonder why a seizure is happening. You don't need to figure out what's causing the seizure. If you know the person has never had a seizure before, call 911.

Plus, the Epilepsy Foundation says to call 911 for seizures if:

- The seizure happened in water
- There is no way to determine the cause of the seizure (ID bracelet, etc.)
- The person is pregnant
- The person has diabetes
- The person is injured
- The seizure lasts more than 5 minutes
- Another seizure happens before the person regains consciousness

Also according to the Epilepsy Foundation, you do *not* need to call 911 if:

- The person is known to have seizures or epilepsy, *and*
- The seizure ended in less than 5 minutes, *and*
- The person wakes up, *and*
- There are no signs of injury, physical distress, or pregnancy

Since it matters whether a seizure lasts longer than 5 minutes, it's important to keep track of how long the shaking and muscle contractions last. Seizures look scary and overwhelming, so use a clock or a watch to time it. Seizures always look like they last longer than they do, even to paramedics.

During a seizure, there's not much you can do to make it stop. Indeed, health care providers often won't try to stop a seizure with medication unless it lasts longer than 10 or 15 minutes. However, there are several things you can do to make the person more comfortable:

- Move hard and sharp objects away from the vicinity of the person if possible
- Loosen any tight clothing around the neck
- Pad under the head with a pillow or a rolled up jacket

Whatever happens, do *not* put anything in the person's mouth. He or she will not swallow his or her tongue and if you put your fingers in his or her mouth, you could get bitten.

After the seizure is finished, the person will slowly begin to wake up. He or she will be groggy and might be confused at first. Try not to bombard him or her with questions. Instead, allow the person to wake up slowly.

Remember, if the seizure lasts more than 5 minutes without stopping or if the person has another seizure right after the first one without waking up, call 911.

Keep an eye on his or her breathing. If he or she is not breathing after the seizure stops, call 911 and start CPR (see Chapter 8).

On the Internet

- www.stroke.org
- www.ninds.nih.gov

19
Breathing Troubles

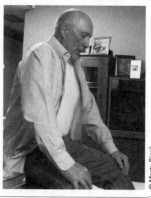

© Marty Bicek

There are only two types of people who get short of breath when they're not exercising: folks who've gotten short of breath before and folks who haven't. First, let's focus on the folks who have never felt short of breath before.

We all know what it means to be out of breath. Running track in high school or a good cardio workout on the treadmill leaves you breathing deep and a little winded. It's not a bad feeling at first and all you have to do is stop the exercise to catch your breath.

The difference when it's a medical condition causing your shortness of breath is that you don't have to exercise to feel that way. You can be sitting on the couch or lying in bed. Maybe you start feeling like you can't breathe while you're having coffee and toast in the morning.

If you know you have a medical condition that causes your shortness of breath—asthma or chronic obstructive pulmonary disease (COPD), for example—you probably know what to do when you start feeling that way. If you've never felt like this before, however, let's ask some questions. This will help us identify a few things that might cause it:

- *Can you bear it?* If you can't handle the feeling, call 911. If you're simply uncomfortable but tolerating this feeling of being out of breath, keep reading.
- *Did your shortness of breath come on suddenly or gradually?* Sudden shortness of breath concerns me more. Heart attacks and blood clots in the lungs can cause shortness of breath to come out of the blue. On the other hand, so can anxiety. All three can also cause chest pain. The trick is to stay calm and call 911 if your shortness of breath came on suddenly without warning. If the shortness of breath came on gradually, we have a few more questions before we call the doctor or 911.

119

- *How long have you had shortness of breath?* After a day or two of shortness of breath, it's time to call the doctor. If you've never had any kind of lung problems in the past, your doctor's likely to tell you to go to the ER or call 911. Regardless, call the doctor first and see what he or she wants you to do.
- *Do you have a cough?* If you are coughing with your shortness of breath, that could indicate fluid, swelling, or mucus in the lungs. If your cough is producing sputum, pay attention to the color and consistency of the sputum. White and frothy means one thing; thick and yellow means another.
- *Do you have a fever or chills?* Fevers indicate infections, and that can tell the doctor (or the paramedics) a lot about what's bothering you. In some areas the ambulance crews don't carry thermometers, so take your own temperature if you think you might have a fever. Another indicator of possible fever is chills: feeling chilly and shivering even when it's not cold in the house.
- *Do you have chest pain?* If you're having chest pain, try to tell if it just hurts to breathe (taking a deep breath or coughing makes it hurt worse) or if the pain is deeper in the chest and doesn't go away or get worse when you breathe. Heart attacks are notorious for causing chest pain, but really bad coughing fits can cause it, too. Indeed, coughing hard enough can even crack ribs in some folks. If you're having chest pain with shortness of breath, go to the ER or call 911. Unless you're absolutely sure your chest pain is from coughing or breathing hard, skip the doctor's office and go right for the ER.
- *Do you have heart, kidney, or liver disease?* Folks who have trouble with their hearts and kidneys can get fluid backed up in the lungs. A telltale sign of backup is swollen ankles. Liver disease can cause abdominal swelling from fluid built up around the liver (ascites). The big belly pushes upward against the diaphragm and the lungs, making it hard to breathe.

Often, with any of these conditions, you'll notice you get winded quickly after just walking to the bathroom or out to pick up the morning paper. If that is happening, call your doctor.

WHAT TO DO FOR SHORTNESS OF BREATH AT HOME

There's not much first aid you can do for trouble breathing. The treatments usually require oxygen, medications, or special equipment (or all three). The best thing is to call your doctor or 911 if you need help.

HOW TO TELL IF SOMEONE IS SHORT OF BREATH

If someone you live with or take care of is complaining of feeling like he or she can't breathe, or feeling short of breath, that's the most important way to tell. Shortness of breath is mostly a feeling, so listening when someone tells you he or she can't breathe is the best way to identify it.

Of course, if he or she can't finish the sentence because he or she is too winded, that's an indicator, too.

There are signs that sort of give away when someone is short of breath, however. One of the most common is pursed lip breathing. When it's hard to exhale (a common problem in sudden shortness of breath) we have a tendency to purse our lips like we're blowing out candles on a birthday cake.

Try it right now: take a deep breath and blow it out. Odds are you pursed your lips. Don't think you did? Okay, try it again, only this time: make an effort not to purse your lips. See how hard it is to push air out when we don't pucker up?

Pursing your lips is just one sign of trouble breathing. The other very common sign (besides being too out of breath to speak) is the way you stand or sit when you're sucking wind. In high school, how did you stand after the coach made you run sprints? (Did your coach call them *wind sprints*? I wonder why.)

I'll bet when you were done running sprints and you were trying to recover, your instinct was to put your hands on your hips or, if you were really out of breath, on your knees. If you're sitting down when you're having trouble breathing, you do the same thing: hands on your knees. It's called the *tripod position.* Like pursed lips and trouble speaking, the tripod position is a good indicator of difficulty breathing.

If you have a medical condition that affects your breathing, your doctor should tell you how to handle bad days when you get more short of breath than usual. As always, if you don't feel like you can handle it, call 911.

There are literally dozens of conditions that can lead to shortness of breath for one reason or another. Some are chronic conditions you just learn to live with (with special tools and medications). Others are short-term diseases that should get better in a few days or maybe weeks. To help you out, I'm going to go over how you should handle the top five respiratory conditions: asthma, COPD, pneumonia, anaphylaxis, and congestive heart failure.

ASTHMA

Asthma is the most common lung disease. It affects airflow through the lungs by producing too much mucus and constricting the airways. Asthma can develop late in life but affects folks of all ages. Chances are, if you have asthma, you already know what to do for your asthma attacks.

Most asthma patients will take a couple of different types of inhaled medication. There are several to choose from and your doctor will most likely have prescribed you one to take every day, regardless of how good or bad you feel, and one to take when you're feeling short of breath.

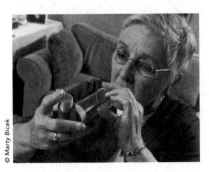

It's important to keep these medications straight. You never want to take the long-acting medicine (the one you take every day no matter what) to try to relieve sudden shortness of breath. Instead, take quick-acting inhalers— sometimes called *rescue inhalers*— when you're feeling short of breath.

If you're unsure of when and how to take your asthma medication—especially regarding which one to take in an emergency—call your doctor and have him or her explain it to you. You can also try asking your pharmacist. This is very important, so don't give up until you fully understand how to take your asthma medicines correctly.

HOW TO USE A RESCUE INHALER

Rescue inhalers, otherwise known as metered dose inhalers, deliver fast-acting medications right into the lungs when you're having trouble breathing. Often, folks get rescue inhalers without learning how to use them correctly. Here are some tips to get the most out of your rescue inhaler:

1. Before you use it, exhale all the way. That's right, blow out every last molecule (I know it's hard to do when you can't breathe, but it's worth it in the end).
2. Close your lips around the mouthpiece and inhale deeply at the same time you squeeze the medicine out. Hold your breath as long as you can.

If you have a spacer (a tube that goes between your lips and the inhaler—see photo above), it's important to use it. Spacers are especially good if you can't hold your breath very long.

COPD

COPD mostly comes from smoking. It can be caused by other things, but those are very rare. There are two specific disorders that lead to COPD; chronic bronchitis and pulmonary emphysema. If you have one, chances are that at least to some degree you also have the other.

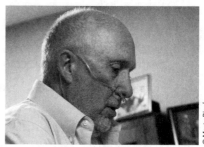

© Marty Bicek

COPD medications are similar to asthma medications (in fact, many COPD patients also have asthma) and the same rules apply. Do not take a long-acting inhaler in the place of a rescue inhaler. Often, folks with COPD have nebulizer machines at home that look, ironically, like smoking pipes. Nebulizers deliver the same medications as handheld inhalers, but in bigger doses over longer periods of time.

Some COPD patients have oxygen at home. The oxygen is delivered through a nasal cannula (a hose for your nose). Your doctor will tell you how much oxygen you can take; it's measured in liters per minute. Usually, COPD patients are allowed to take a maximum of 2 liters per minute, but there are exceptions. Be sure to ask your doctor if you can have more oxygen when you're feeling especially short of breath.

ANAPHYLAXIS (ALLERGIC REACTION)

Allergies usually affect the skin. They cause itching, redness, hives, and swelling. However some allergies can affect the lungs, causing very rapid reactions with narrowing of the airways, coughing, and sneezing. When an allergy affects breathing, we call it *anaphylaxis*. Besides breathing, anaphylaxis can also lead to a dangerously low blood pressure.

Those who are prone to anaphylaxis usually know what they are deathly allergic to. Some of the most common allergies include peanuts, eggs, latex, and bee stings. There are just too many to list here. If you are allergic to something that causes very severe reactions (or if you already know for sure you get anaphylactic reactions), you should be carrying an epinephrine auto-injector (EpiPen is the most common brand name).

Epinephrine is basically the same as adrenaline, the hormone responsible for that rush you get when you jump out of an airplane on your 80th birthday—or when you lean back too far in a chair and almost fall over but catch yourself. Epinephrine does an incredible job of reversing anaphylaxis.

HOW TO USE AN EPIPEN

Epinephrine auto-injectors come in a variety of styles, but the EpiPen is the most common and all auto-injectors work in a similar fashion.

1. Unscrew the yellow cap from the container and take out the EpiPen.
2. Make sure the contents of the EpiPen are clear and not yellow. Yellow coloring means the drug is not safe to use.
3. Take off the gray cap on the back of the EpiPen.
4. Press the EpiPen firmly into the thigh (right through any clothes) and hold it in place for 10 seconds.
5. With one hand, put the used EpiPen back into the container it came in and put the yellow cap back on.

If you have to use an EpiPen, you need to call 911 unless your doctor gave you some other instructions. When the ambulance arrives, you can give the used EpiPen to the paramedics. They have a special container for used syringes and needles.

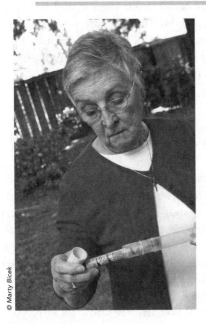

© Marty Bicek

The other drug that works really well for anaphylaxis is Benadryl (diphenhydramine), the same drug you take for hay fever or to help you sleep sometimes. Epinephrine reverses an anaphylactic reaction, but Benadryl stops it from developing—or after the epinephrine, Benadryl keeps the anaphylaxis from returning.

Anaphylaxis isn't as simple as taking a little epinephrine to make it all better, however, so even if you take a shot of epinephrine and down a couple Benadryls, you still need to go to the hospital. Often, doctors will also treat anaphylaxis patients with corticosteroids to help them recover, which may take several days.

PULMONARY EDEMA

Congestive heart failure (CHF) happens when one side of the heart isn't pumping as efficiently as the other side. CHF can result in the lungs filling up with fluid, also known as *pulmonary edema*. Besides CHF, folks with kidney failure who need dialysis can suffer from pulmonary edema if they don't get their dialysis on a regular basis.

For kidney failure patients the treatment is simple: get dialysis. In most cases that will require a call to your doctor or maybe directly to 911 for a ride to the hospital.

For patients with CHF, pulmonary edema indicates a need to decrease how hard the heart is working to pump blood. Sometimes, your doctor may prescribe nitroglycerin for this. In other cases, you'll just need to go to the hospital. Either way, if you're prone to this sort of thing, you probably already take a water pill to get rid of excess fluid.

People with CHF, especially those on water pills, know that if their CHF is getting worse or if they skipped a water pill, their ankles swell up. Suffice it to say that if your ankles are swollen (filled with water), your lungs are filled with water, too.

Pneumonia

Pneumonia is a type of lung inflammation that results in mucus or fluid building up in the lungs and airways. It usually comes on from an infection, which can start anywhere. Pneumonia most commonly comes with other signs and symptoms, like fever, chills, or cough. Pneumonia can come on all by itself or after some other infection like the flu.

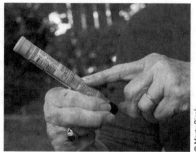
© Marty Bicek

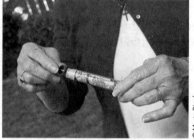
© Marty Bicek

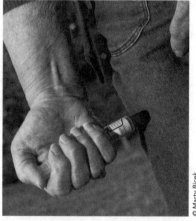
© Marty Bicek

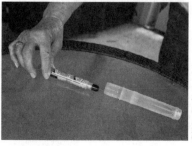
© Marty Bicek

Sometimes, pneumonia can happen from accidentally getting food or liquid down the windpipe (called *aspiration pneumonia*). Often this will lead to an infection. Aspiration pneumonia is common in people who have a hard time swallowing, such as those with traumatic brain injuries or strokes.

Pneumonia can't really be treated at home. This is a condition for which you'll have to go to the doctor or to the hospital. Depending on the type of infection, you may need to take medications.

ON THE INTERNET

- firstaid.about.com/od/shortnessofbreat1
- www.nlm.nih.gov/medlineplus/breathingproblems.html

20

Is That Chest Pain, or Is Someone Sitting on My Chest?

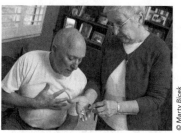
© Marty Bicek

L et's get the important stuff out of the way first. Are you having chest pain or pressure? If you are, ask yourself these questions:

- Can I make it feel better or worse by moving or pressing on my chest?
- Does it hurt to cough or breathe?
- Have I ever felt this before?

If you answer "no" to all three questions, put down this book and call 911. If you can answer yes to some or all of these, I still have one more question for you: Do you think the chest pain might be from your heart? If the answer is yes, call 911. Later, you can come back and read this chapter to find out why you needed to rush.

Heart attacks come in all shapes and sizes. There's been a lot of coverage in the media about heart attacks and symptoms of heart attacks. One of the things we've learned over the years is that heart attack symptoms can be all kinds of different things: pain, pressure, shortness of breath, burning, arm pain, neck pain, jaw pain, cold sweats, or even just nausea.

With all of those "new" symptoms we've discovered, I'm afraid the most obvious one has kind of been lost in the noise: chest pain. Chest pain is still the most common symptom of a heart attack. So if you have chest pain and you think it might be your heart, call 911 immediately.

When Chest Pain Makes a Paramedic Nervous

Not all chest pain is the same. Have you ever pulled a muscle lifting something heavy? Have you ever had sore ribs after coughing for days, or how about after vomiting for hours from food poisoning? That kind of chest pain is in the muscles between your ribs. It hurts, but it won't kill you.

Lung infections will sometimes irritate the lining between the lungs and the inside of the chest. The lining gets dry and irritated. When that happens it's called *pleurisy*, and it hurts really, really bad to breathe.

Chest pain coming from your heart is different. It's deep. It doesn't get any better when you massage it or take shallow breaths. It doesn't get suddenly worse when you laugh or cough. It doesn't feel sore; it feels scary.

The heart is a muscle just like the muscles that live between your ribs or move your arms or allow you to walk. When the heart muscle is straining, starving, or damaged, it hurts, just like any other muscle in your body would hurt. I suppose if you could touch your heart when it was hurting, you could make it hurt worse (or make it feel better). Because you can't touch it, you can't really change the pain it feels.

When the heart hurts it's being damaged. If it continues to be damaged for too long, the muscle dies (a heart attack). If too much heart muscle dies, then it can't pump blood any longer and the heart-attack person dies.

When a person calls 911 complaining of chest pain, the paramedics are going to ask a series of questions. The answers to those questions help us decide if we're going to worry about this chest pain being a heart attack or not.

- *How did the pain start?* We want to know if the pain came on suddenly or gradually over time. Heart attacks come from a blockage—usually a blood clot—restricting blood flow to the heart muscle. As soon as the clot gets stuck, the pain starts—suddenly.
- *Does anything make the pain better?* Heart muscle pain is deep in the chest where movement and breathing aren't going to make much difference on how much worse or better the pain is getting.
- *What does the pain feel like?* Many of my patients think this is a silly question. "It hurts, idiot" is a common response. However, this is one of the most important questions we ask. We're asking our victims to describe the pain. Is it an ache or a sharp, stabbing pain? Does it feel like pressure or squeezing? Depending on the description of the pain, the paramedic might begin to suspect a heart attack. The most common description of heart-related chest pain is pressure or squeezing in the chest. Sometimes, it's described as suffocating or not being able to take a deep breath. Heart pain doesn't have to be pressure, but if pressure is described, I get nervous.
- *Does the pain go anywhere else?* Heart-related chest pain has a habit of spreading (we call it *radiating*) from the chest out to other parts, namely down the left arm or up into the neck and jaw. Sometimes it radiates to the back. It doesn't have to radiate anywhere, or it can go off in some wild direction, but if it goes to the left arm or the jaw, we paramedics get nervous again.

- *How bad is it?* By now, you've probably run into the pain scale. It's the health care industry's way of trying to apply a number to everything. The pain scale is a number from 1 to 10. A tiny little bit of pain, almost nothing at all, is a 1. The worst pain you've ever felt (ladies usually chalk that one up to childbirth) is a 10. The higher the number, the more concerned we get.
- *How long have you had the pain?* Here's a super important question, because the longer a heart attack goes untreated, the more heart muscle dies. When heart muscle dies, it's permanent. We want to get heart attacks fixed as quickly as possible to save as much muscle as we can. Our saying is: *time is muscle.*

If someone calls 911 with chest pressure that started suddenly an hour ago, radiates to the left arm, is 8 on a scale of 1 to 10, and no matter what position he or she sits in, he or she can't get comfortable, I'm going to assume he or she is having a heart attack until proven otherwise. What he or she may or may not know is that calling 911 is the absolute best thing he or she could do.

Never Go to the Doctor With Chest Pain

Always call 911 when you have chest pain. If for some reason you insist on getting in the car and going somewhere, don't. Don't go to the doctor's office—drive to the emergency room (better yet, pull over and call 911).

If you're having a heart attack, your doctor doesn't have the tools you need to fix it.

I know it feels like every time you go to the ER the wait is horrendous. I know it seems like the best place to go is to the doctor's office because you get personal care from your doctor. Maybe it costs you more to go to the ER because your insurance co-pay is cheaper for an office visit.

If you go to the doctor's office and tell the doctor you are having chest pain, the doctor will call an ambulance for you. More than likely, the doctor won't want the ambulance to show up at the office with lights and sirens, so he or she will tell the ambulance team not to make any fuss. If the ambulance is driving to your emergency without lights on and another emergency happens, it will be sent to the other emergency instead and you'll have to wait longer.

If, on the other hand, you call 911 from your home, the ambulance will be dispatched with lights and sirens and, no matter what, it will come to your house.

The difference doesn't end there. Your doctor might be able to check your heart with an EKG, and he or she can probably give you some nitroglycerin and aspirin, but if you're having a heart attack you need a procedure to clear the blood clot and get blood flowing again. The longer you go without that procedure, the more chance there is that you won't recover from your heart attack.

Heart attacks need to be treated right away, and the most important treatment can't be done in an ambulance or in the doctor's office. Emergency departments have plans in place to quickly get heart-attack victims into the procedure room and fix the heart attack before it creates too much damage.

Skip the doctor's office and call 911 from home if you feel chest pain and think it might be your heart. An ambulance will respond immediately. The crew will treat your pain and start screening you for the procedure on the way to the hospital. The emergency room physician will decide if you need to be treated right away, and the hospital staff will take you directly to the procedure room if they need to.

WHAT TO DO IF YOU HAVE CHEST PAIN

The 911 operator will advise you on what to do as you wait for the ambulance. If you're having chest pain, the 911 operator might tell you to take an aspirin. There has been a lot of stuff on TV and in magazines about taking aspirin if you think you're having a heart attack, so let me clear some things up.

Aspirin will not cure a heart attack. The purpose of aspirin is to thin the blood a little and cut down on the inflamed blood vessels and muscles in the heart. Aspirin is not a bad thing to take if you think it's your heart causing the chest pain, but it's not enough by itself.

Aspirin should only come *after* you've called 911. Don't delay calling an ambulance in order to take an aspirin. If you don't get around to taking an aspirin before the ambulance gets there, that's okay. The paramedic will probably give you some aspirin anyway.

OTHER DRUGS FOR CHEST PAIN

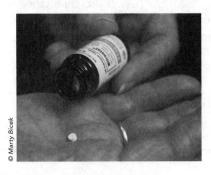

Aspirin isn't the only medication to take when you're having chest pain. If you've had chest pains before, you might have a prescription for nitroglycerin (the little white pill that goes under your tongue). Nitroglycerin opens up the blood vessels carrying blood to the heart and makes it easier for the heart to do its job.

JONATHON'S GRANDPA: WHY YOU DON'T DRIVE WHEN YOU HAVE CHEST PAIN

Ed was a 65-year-old retiree. He was a former Marine and a devoted grandfather who spent his summer weekdays with his 8-year-old grandson, Jonathon. Jonathon's mom and dad both worked, so Ed was the go-to guy when school was out.

I met Ed after he pulled into the local fire station. He was on his way to the hospital and stopped at the firehouse to ask directions. The department's office manager took one look at Ed's sweaty, pale face and called an ambulance—us.

When we got there, the first thing my partner and I noticed was that Ed was gray and dripping sweat. He complained of chest pressure that had been getting worse all morning. He tried to drive himself to the hospital but couldn't remember how to get there.

We loaded Ed up quickly and were ready to go when he told us that his grandson was with him. Jonathon was standing behind the counter in the office, so I'd assumed he was the office manager's son. Jonathon couldn't be left behind, so he hopped into the back of the ambulance with Ed and me.

As we headed to the hospital, I put Ed on the heart monitor and checked his blood pressure. I chatted with Jonathon while I gave Ed oxygen, aspirin, and nitroglycerin. I also started an intravenous line.

I was giving the report over the radio to the emergency department when Ed's heart stopped. We were on the freeway. If Ed had been driving with Jonathon in the pickup truck—as he had been before stopping at the firehouse—they surely would have crashed. Ed would have died and Jonathon might have as well.

As it turned out, Ed's heart started after a quick shock and a little CPR. Jonathon was a trooper about the whole thing and didn't shed a tear until after we got to the hospital.

Several months later I ran into Ed and Jonathon. Ed gave me a hug and Jonathon let me know that he was really scared (he also told me that when he grows up, he's going to be a Marine).

Nitroglycerin has been around for many years and is a very important tool for treating heart attacks. It is not without its dangers, however. Here are a couple of things you should know about nitroglycerin:

- Don't take nitroglycerin if you've taken Viagra or any other erectile dysfunction drug in the last 48 hours, and be sure to tell any paramedics or nurses that you've used those drugs. Nitroglycerin lowers blood pressure and erectile dysfunction drugs do, too; together they can lower your blood pressure enough to cause your heart to stop.
- Because nitroglycerin lowers your blood pressure, you might feel flushed or weak after taking it. Don't try to stand or walk if you get this feeling—you might pass out and fall.
- Nitroglycerin is very volatile. It's the same substance used to make dynamite. It isn't going to blow up if you drop the bottle, but it goes bad very quickly when exposed to air and light. Keep it bottled up and out of direct light as much as possible. When your nitroglycerin expires, get a new bottle.

On the Internet

- www.nlm.nih.gov/medlineplus/chestpain.html
- firstaid.about.com/od/heartattacks

21

Abdominal Pains and Lower Back Pain

B ellyaches are almost never diagnosed. There's just so much going on in your abdomen, and it differs between women and the men. Abdominal pain is the great mystery of the emergency department.

There are some pretty common pains that I'll cover here, but the most important thing to remember is to trust your gut (no pun intended). If you think your abdominal pain is something serious enough to need an ambulance, put down the book and call 911. If you think it's bad enough to see the doctor—but you don't need the ER—then call your doctor and make an appointment.

Paramedics go through a priority checklist when we hear you complaining of abdominal pain that we can't blame on something obvious (like getting punched in the gut). First, is the pain coming from above the belly button? If it is above the belly button, then does it feel like aching or pressure? If so, does it travel (we call that *radiate*) to your arm or jaw?

If you have abdominal pain that meets all three criteria, then call 911. It's hard to tell where the chest ends and the abdomen begins, so pain above the belly button is often treated like chest pain (see Chapter 20).

PANCREATITIS

Pancreatitis can affect anyone and can cause pain in the same area; above the belly button. Pancreatitis can be a sudden infection or it can be from a chronic condition that just keeps cropping up.

GALL BLADDERS AND GALL STONES

If you're a woman over the age of 40, especially if you have a fair complexion and a few extra pounds (I'm not saying you do), then sharp or burning pain right between your belly button and your breastbone might be related to your gall bladder. Depending on the type of gall bladder issue creating the pain, you could have cramping pain there as well.

APPENDICITIS

The appendix is a little pouch that hangs off the beginning of your large colon. It holds bacteria that we use to digest food. Sometimes it can get blocked and become infected, which is known as *appendicitis.*

In most cases, appendicitis causes abdominal pain in the lower right abdomen (see the following for more on areas of the abdomen). However, as the appendix gets more inflamed, it can burst and cause a more widespread infection of the abdominal wall (see *Peritonitis*). If that happens, you might feel a little better at first, then start feeling pain again, along with fever, chills, and a swollen abdomen.

DIVERTICULITIS

Diverticulosis is a condition that becomes more common as we get older and more common if we get constipation a lot. Diverticula are little bulges that happen in the intestines from years of use. Sometimes those little bulges can get infected and that's known as *diverticulitis.*

Diverticulitis will almost certainly cause abdominal pain and can also have fever, chills, vomiting, or diarrhea. If the infection gets bad enough, the intestines can rupture and allow fecal matter into the abdomen (similar to the worst-case scenario of appendicitis).

PERITONITIS

The lining of the abdomen is called the peritoneum. Inflammation of the peritoneum is known as *peritonitis* and just might be the most painful of all abdominal infections. Peritonitis usually comes with abdominal pain from all over the abdomen with fever, chills, and vomiting. Peritonitis may also cause abdominal swelling and a tight or hard abdomen, not to mention the abdomen may be extremely tender to touch.

KIDNEY STONES

Kidney stones come from calcium buildup in the kidneys—kind of like that white, crusty stuff that builds up in your kitchen pipes after a few years. Kidney stones are a common cause of excruciating lower abdominal pain. We look for the pain to start on one side or the other at what is known as the *flank*, on the back where the kidneys are located. If you were a car, the spot on your body that we call the flank would be your blind spot on the freeway.

Kidney stones cause extra bad pain that comes in waves and gets much worse when you try to pee. They will bring the toughest among us to tears. I recommend a trip to the emergency department in that case for some well-deserved pain control.

GASTROENTERITIS

Gastroenteritis is probably the most common abdominal issue of all. You might call it the "stomach flu" or "food poisoning." Neither is really correct, but they're both close enough. Most cases of gastroenteritis are from bacteria that we get from consuming contaminated food or fluids. We get nausea, vomiting, abdominal pain and cramping, and usually diarrhea. We can also get a fever and body aches.

Pain below your belly button can be from many things including appendicitis, bowel obstructions, and urinary tract infections (UTIs; in women). Constipation is a side effect of several common medications—including opioid pain medications like Vicodin and Oxycontin. Constipation can lead to a bowel obstruction, which may become an infection.

UTIs can also cause abdominal pain in women. In men, UTIs commonly cause rectal pain. In both sexes, UTIs can cause decreased urine and pain or burning when urinating. They can also cause fevers and fatigue like any other infection (see Chapter 23 for more on infections).

Truly figuring out what is causing abdominal pain requires looking at all the symptoms. These are the symptoms that paramedics look for to rule out the most common conditions:

- Vomiting
- Diarrhea
- Fever
- Body aches
- Fatigue

- Dizziness
- Trouble urinating
- Swollen abdomen
- Hard abdomen
- No bowel movements

To make abdominal pain easier to describe, we have to split it up. Draw a big, imaginary plus sign right in the middle of your abdomen with the lines crossing at your belly button. That divides your abdomen into four parts (called *quadrants*): right upper, right lower, left upper, and left lower. Paramedics suspect different types of problems depending in which area you say the pain is.

- *Right Upper Abdominal Quadrant:* The liver lives here. If you are hurting in this quadrant, there can be a problem with the liver. We're especially concerned if it starts to swell or gets very tender to the touch. Sometimes a hiatal hernia can cause upper abdominal pain (either side) as well.
- *Right Lower Abdominal Quadrant:* The infamous appendix lies in the lower right quadrant. Pain and tenderness there (if you still have an appendix) is cause for concern, especially if you've been running a fever and had vomiting, constipation, or diarrhea. To muddy the waters a little, we're more concerned with appendicitis if you have pain in this area, but the appendix is notorious for causing pain in other areas of the abdomen also.
- *Left Upper Abdominal Quadrant:* The spleen is found in the left upper quadrant and usually behaves unless it's kicked by a cow or suffers some other unhappy event. In some cases it can swell or become infected.
- *Left Lower Abdominal Quadrant:* Your aorta, the largest artery in your body, runs through the left side of your belly. Any severe pain to the left of your belly button (upper or lower quadrant) can be a weak spot in the aorta (called an *abdominal aortic aneurysm*).

LOWER BACK PAIN

Doctors look differently at back pain that's been going on for more than 6 weeks (called *chronic back pain*) and new back pain that's been there for less than 6 weeks. This book is focused on urgent problems, rather than long-term ones. I'm going to assume if you've had back pain for more than 6 weeks that you've at least contacted your doctor. Hopefully, you and your doctor have worked out a plan to help you feel better. If that's the case, then you should call your doctor if your pain is getting worse.

On the other hand, if you don't usually have back pain and now you do, there are some things you should know:

- *The good news:* Lower back pain usually starts feeling better within a couple of weeks and is much better (if not completely gone) within 4 to 6 weeks.
- *The bad news:* Once you get lower back pain the first time, you're likely to suffer from it again.

As long as each episode of back pain feels about the same, you can expect your recovery to go about the same as well (if it took 4 weeks the first time, it will probably take 4 weeks the second time). If the pain is totally different, consider it something new and read the following directions.[5]

There are some things you can do for lower back pain at home, but before I go into those things, let's look at who to call (the ambulance or the doctor's office).

Get to the ER—either have someone drive you or call 911 for an ambulance—if you have any of the following with your back pain:

- Trouble controlling your bladder or bowels (incontinence)
- Unable to urinate or have a bowel movement (urine retention or constipation)
- Both legs are suddenly weak (not just one)
- Numbness in your groin or "saddle" area (the parts that come in contact with a bicycle seat)

If you're older than 50 (most folks reading this book will be in that category), you should call your doctor for any new feeling of lower back pain. It may be several days before your doctor will get you in. You should also call your doctor to make an appointment if you have any of these other symptoms along with your back pain:

- Fever for more than a day or two
- Really bad pain at night or at rest that affects your sleep or doesn't allow you to find a comfortable position, at least for a while
- Back pain is gradually getting worse
- Gradual numbness or weakness in one or both legs
- You were exerting yourself recently (lifting, digging, twisting, etc.)
- Losing weight without a reason (over 10 pounds in 6 months or less)
- You've had cancer

While you're waiting for an appointment (or waiting for the pain to go away), you can do some things to help make your back pain more manageable. Your best bet is to stay active. Don't crawl in bed and stay there, or your back pain is likely to get worse. Modify your activity just enough to keep the pain from spreading out from your lower back to your shoulders, legs, and arms. Stay away from:

- Bed rest
- Sitting for long periods
- Heavy lifting
- Bending over or twisting your back, especially while lifting

To control the pain, you can try a couple of things: over-the-counter pain medications and ice or heat. Whether you prefer ice or heat is up to you, but neither should be left in place for more than 20 minutes. Never put ice directly on the skin or it could cause frostbite.

Pain medications should be limited to the least amount you can take to make the pain bearable and never exceed the maximum dose on the label. Most doctors agree that ibuprofen (Advil or Motrin) is best for muscle pain, but sometimes I get better relief with acetaminophen (Tylenol). Don't try to make pain go away completely, just try to make it tolerable. It will get better eventually.

On the Internet

- www.nlm.nih.gov/medlineplus/ency/article/003120.htm
- firstaid.about.com/od/firstaidbasics/qt/06_abdpain.htm

22

Feeling Faint

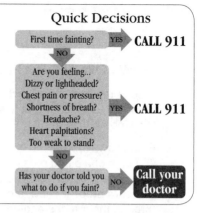

Quick Decisions

First time fainting? **YES** → **CALL 911**

NO ↓

Are you feeling...
Dizzy or lightheaded?
Chest pain or pressure?
Shortness of breath?
Headache?
Heart palpitations?
Too weak to stand?   **YES** → **CALL 911**

NO ↓

Has your doctor told you
what to do if you faint?   NO → **Call your doctor**

F ainting is the same as passing out. It's a loss of consciousness that happens with little or no warning. When you pass out and wake up all by yourself a few seconds or minutes later, medical folks like me call it *syncope*.

If someone around you has just fainted and hasn't woken up yet, call 911 immediately. If that person isn't breathing, start CPR (Chapter 8).

A lot of fainting follows a common pattern. People who faint describe first feeling flushed or hot, followed by their knees buckling, and waking up on the floor. If you see someone faint, you'll notice him or her go limp and collapse. Most of the time, he or she will break out in a sweat when he or she faints or right before. In most cases of fainting, the person will wake up in a few moments.

Lots of things can cause fainting. The most common cause is a sensitive vagus nerve. The vagus nerve is a direct line to the brain that runs all the way through our digestive systems, from the mouth to the anus. When the vagus nerve is stimulated (like when we have to poop), it sends a signal to the brain to decrease blood pressure and slow the heart down. This kind of fainting is almost like a reflex.

The loss of blood pressure is so severe in some folks that they pass out (see the sidebar, *How Low Blood Pressure Makes Us Pass Out*).

People who have syncope from an overactive vagus nerve (called *vasovagal syncope*) often have it all their lives. The fainting from lifelong vasovagal syncope will usually start around puberty. Syncope isn't particularly dangerous, as long as they have the good fortune not to faint while they're climbing a mountain or driving a car.

Vasovagal syncope is just one kind of fainting. There are also other, more dangerous types of fainting. Taking care of a person who has fainted is a little bit about making sure he or she is okay right now, but also figuring out why he or she fainted in the first place.

HOW LOW BLOOD PRESSURE MAKES US PASS OUT

Blood pressure has a function. We always hear about high blood pressure being bad, which is true, but how often do we hear about low blood pressure?

Blood flows around the body precisely *because* it's under pressure. Too high of a blood pressure puts extra stress on the walls of the arteries and veins, which leads to damage over time. When blood pressure drops too low, there isn't enough force to move blood through the arteries and get oxygen to important organs and tissues.

Three things have to work together to regulate blood pressure: heart rate (how fast the heart beats), how much blood is in the body, and how tightly the arteries are squeezing. If we lose too much blood (through bleeding or dehydration), our blood pressure drops. If our arteries get loose and stop squeezing or if our hearts beat too slow, our blood pressure drops.

The most important organ to fill with blood is the brain. It also happens to be at the top of the body, which means there has to be enough blood pressure to fight gravity in order to get all the way up there. If our blood pressure drops too much to get blood all the way up to the brain, we can pass out.

DEHYDRATION AND SHOCK

We need water to make blood. When we don't have enough water, we don't have enough blood and we don't have enough blood pressure. Stimulating the vagus nerve when the system is already a quart or two low makes things that much worse.

Several conditions cause dehydration. Vomiting, diarrhea, heat illness, burns, and infections are just some of the things that can lead to dehydration. Vomiting and diarrhea also stimulate the vagus nerve—I think that qualifies as a double whammy.

Being low on blood volume can also be from direct loss, otherwise known as bleeding. Severe bleeding—and severe dehydration for that matter—can lead to a condition known as shock. Shock happens when the blood pressure is low enough to be life-threatening. A person who passes out from shock is much different than a person who passes out from syncope.

If the person passed out following a significant injury, assume he or she is bleeding. If the person passed out while exhibiting signs of heat illness (Chapter 24), assume it's heatstroke, a life-threatening illness.

Shock can also come from a severe allergic reaction, known as anaphylactic shock. If you suspect anaphylactic shock, you should call 911 immediately and help the person with his or her epinephrine injector if he or she has one (Chapter 19).

Psychological Triggers

Some folks stimulate the vagus nerve when they panic or get scared. Do you get weak in the knees when you see blood? My wife says she used to get a little woozy when she saw blood—even passed out in high school once during a health film (she's an EMT now).

When I directed the EMS program at the community college, I had a few students pass out while watching procedures in the emergency room. Nobody got hurt (even those who fell in the ER) and everybody turned out just fine. Psychological fainting isn't an emergency.

Drugs or Alcohol

Drinking too much alcohol makes me pass out—you're probably the same way. It's not fainting, but it is definitely passing out. Alcohol also makes us dehydrated. Alcohol has a diuretic effect; in other words, it makes us pee. As if making you feel fuzzy and making you pee wasn't enough, alcohol also loosens up those arteries and makes it harder for your body to maintain blood pressure.

You can die from drinking too much alcohol, but that's usually a younger person's problem. I'm going to go out on a limb here, but most readers of this book have probably learned a lesson or two about how much alcohol they can comfortably consume. However, if someone around you has consumed more than his or her fair share of tequila and won't wake up, it's time to call 911.

Plenty of drugs of all kinds—over the counter, behind the counter, prescription, and street corner drugs—can lead you to unconsciousness. It's not fainting, but it can be dangerous. Some drugs affect the brain directly, while others mess with the heart, lower blood pressure, or lead to dehydration. Some drugs do all of these things. Here are some of the drugs most likely to affect our ability to stay vertical:

- Nitrates make the blood pressure drop quickly
- Erectile dysfunction drugs can lower blood pressure
- Nitrates and erectile dysfunction drugs together can drop blood pressure to life-threateningly low levels
- Diuretics make you urinate more often, leading to dehydration
- Opioids (narcotic pain relievers) lower blood pressure and slow breathing
- Heart medications might slow the heart rate and lower blood pressure
- Blood pressure drugs lower blood pressure, which is what they're meant to do

PAIN

Similar to a psychological trigger, pain can stimulate the vagus nerve and lead to syncope. Some folks pass out from getting stuck with a needle. Other people can drop like flies from stubbing a toe or breaking a finger.

The problem with writing off fainting as being related to pain is that serious injuries are also often painful. It would be bad to assume someone has passed out from the pain of getting conked on the noggin just to find out he or she really has a concussion (Chapter 14).

HEART

Heart-related syncope is pretty dangerous stuff. The heart is the pump for your whole blood flow system. When it works correctly, everything is fine, but when it malfunctions, blood pressure can drop. When it fails, blood pressure can drop and never come back.

There are several things that can go wrong with the heart and lead to passing out:

- It can beat too fast
- It can beat too slow
- It can beat irregularly
- It can be too weak

During a heart attack, the heart can do any of the things on this list. However, you don't have to have a heart attack for any of these to happen.

There are some warning signs to look for when someone faints to make us worry about the heart. Chest pain or pressure, shortness of breath, and palpitations are all signs that the fainting might have been because the heart is not doing what it should. Anyone with these symptoms before or after fainting should get an ambulance.

SIGNS AND SYMPTOMS OF FAINTING

Fainting is passing out, but there are other symptoms and signs that can be associated with it:

- Dizziness or feeling light-headed
- Flushed or pale color
- Confusion
- Nausea
- Sweating
- Weakness
- Feeling hot
- Trembling or shaking (not a seizure, however)
- Tunnel vision or blurred vision
- Sudden trouble hearing
- Eye shaking (nystagmus)
- Headache
- Shortness of breath
- Loss of bowel or bladder control (incontinence)

Lots of folks complain about fainting right before or right after having a bowel movement. That makes sense if you think about it, because the vagus nerve runs through the entire digestive tract. Some folks even pass out after experiencing abdominal cramps.

WHAT TO EXPECT

Fainting can range from very subtle to quite violent, depending on who's fainting and how. In the movies, the leading lady always puts a hand to her forehead before falling gracefully into the arms of her leading man. In real life, blood is draining from the brain and the brain is not going to like that very much.

Most of the time the brain just shuts down. Muscles don't get the messages they need to stay upright and the whole mess (arms, legs, torso, and head) just collapses into a heap. Sometimes we fall forward. Sometimes we fall backward. If we're sitting, we might slump into our chair or roll out of it.

Once in a while, the brain has a little fit. It doesn't like draining blood after all. It tries to hang on and a bit of noise goes out over the communication lines like static on the phone. That noise makes the muscles twitch a bit, sometimes a lot. It can even look like a very short seizure.

Growing up far out of town with our party line telephones, every once in a while a car would hit a telephone pole. The surge of noise it created would cause our phone to ring for just a second—not even a whole ring. It's the same thing in the nervous system when the brain drains, except the "ring" is more of a shudder.

In fact, you've probably had a little party line ring of your own. You know that twitch some people get when they're falling asleep (it drives my wife nuts when I do it)? That twitch is known as a myoclonic jerk and it's really common when we're going from conscious to unconscious.

AFTER FAINTING

My mom used to have one of those little drinking birds that had water in it. When it was up, the water would drain one way and make it dip, then drain the other and lift it up again.

Our bodies work very much the same way when we pass out from syncope. The blood drains from our brains and makes us lose consciousness, but as soon as we land flat, our blood starts filling back into the brain and wakes us up. Depending on who you are and why you passed out, you can recover very quickly or very slowly.

Generally, here's what happens:

- Sweating dries up
- Color returns
- Heart beat speeds up, sometimes very fast

Fainting isn't dangerous, but sudden cardiac arrest is deadly. Unfortunately, at first they look exactly the same. It's really important that if breathing stops, you must call 911 and start CPR (Chapter 8).

FAINTING TREATMENT

If this is the first time the person has ever fainted, it's time to call 911. There are so many causes of fainting and some of them are very dangerous. There's absolutely no way to tell what's causing the fainting without a trip to the emergency department.

If you don't know whether the person has ever fainted before, then call 911. It's better to err on the side of overdoing it than it is to wait too long. Besides, if he or she wakes up in the meantime and tells the ambulance thanks but no thanks, no harm done. Even if you know he or she has a history of fainting, if he or she doesn't wake up after 3 or 4 minutes, call 911 anyway.

Once someone has fainted, whether you're going to call 911 or not, you need to keep an eye on his or her breathing. If he or she fell into a weird position—especially if the neck is bent—try to lay him or her flat on the ground, either on his or her back or side. If you want to speed recovery, you can try elevating his or her feet, but it probably won't change anything.

PREVENTING FAINTING

You might not be able to do anything to prevent fainting, but sometimes you can avoid it if you feel it approaching. If you suffer from syncope, you probably know how it feels as it's coming on.

When you feel that flushed feeling or the woozy dizziness, lie down. That's the body's way of making things better after you faint, so you can get a jump on recovery by lying down first. And if it doesn't work, at least you can't fall very far. If you can't lie down, whatever you do, don't stand up.

Don't get dehydrated. Drink plenty of fluids (see *How Much Water is Enough?* in Chapter 24).

ON THE INTERNET

- www.mayoclinic.com/health/first-aid-fainting/FA00052
- firstaid.about.com/od/chronicillnesses/qt/08_Fainting.htm

23
Infections and Fevers

We all get sick. You can be old or young and get a fever. When we think of fevers, we tend to think of kids staying home from school with an ice pack on their noggins and thermometers in their mouths. Maybe we even think of childhood diseases like chicken pox or scarlet fever.

By the time you get old enough to pay taxes, fevers were more of an annoyance than an excuse to play hooky. Most of us can't afford to take a day off just because we get a case of the chills or a stuffy nose. As an adult, we think of fevers as costing us money and making it awfully hard just to get through the day.

The problem with us adults is that sometimes we don't take fevers seriously enough. A fever is the immune system doing its job, so why worry? It'll go away soon.

As we age, however, the cells and tissues that make up our immune systems don't work as well. Think of your immune system as an army, waiting to battle intruders—germs—that invade to make you sick. As the battles rage, you get hot. The bigger the battle, the hotter it gets.

It takes lots of firepower on both sides of this war to really heat things up. When your immune system gets weaker, your fevers aren't as high, even if you have a serious infection.[6]

Likewise, when your immune system is a bit weaker, the infection is allowed to grow and get stronger. The problem is you don't know you have an infection at first because what has traditionally been the best indicator of infection—a fever—isn't happening. Once the infection gets stronger, either your immune system is finally mobilized enough to give you a higher body temperature, or else the infection is winning.[7]

Because we can't rely on fever as the major telltale sign of an infection, we have to look at other things. One of the more common complaints I get in the ambulance from my older patients is simply weakness. Another is fatigue. These are the types of things people call on when they know in their gut that what's going on with them is worse than any specific symptom. In other words, they call me out because they just don't feel good.

NORMAL BODY TEMPERATURE AIN'T WHAT IT USED TO BE

Normal body temperature taken under the tongue is 98.6°F, plus or minus a degree. For those of you who take your temperature with the metric system, that's 37°C .

As we age and become less active, our normal body temperatures get lower, but how much lower is different for each person. Your normal body temperature may not be the same as your spouse's, even if you're the same age.

Also as we age, our ability to generate fevers becomes weaker. By the time an older adult's temperature goes up enough to be considered a "fever," the infection may have become very serious.

What does this mean for you? Well, you could have an infection even if you don't have a fever and if you do get a fever—no matter how small—call the doctor.

Anything that hinders you from doing your daily routine is potentially a medical symptom. Are you falling more often? Dizzy? Having trouble concentrating or remembering? Infections can cause all of these and more. Worse, you could get pretty sick long before you ever develop a fever.

As I was writing this chapter, I was called to pick up a patient from a nursing home (literally as I was writing it—I had my laptop computer with me in the ambulance). The patient was able to chat with us but had not had an appetite and her blood tests had just been completed. It turns out she had valley fever (an infection common in northern California).

Her temperature was 97.9°F; lower than normal.

Now that we know almost anything can be an infection—fever or not—let's look at some of the more common infections I see in my older patients.

THE FLU

Influenza, the notorious virus that comes around every year; a wolf in sheep's clothing pretending to be any number of lame head colds or sinus infection. The flu sneaks up on you and knocks you down when you least expect it (kind of like the "cow tipping" I used to do growing up—except that now I'm the cow and flu is the punk teenager who really needs a summer job).

Probably the most misunderstood thing about the flu is what it is. Lots of folks believe the flu is a disease of the gut, causing you to throw up and develop a bout of diarrhea.

Nope. The flu is all respiratory. It affects the lungs, causing trouble breathing and serious coughing. The flu might lead to vomiting eventually, but it's really a problem with the lungs and that's why it leads to pneumonia.

According to the CDC, here are the symptoms of the regular, garden-variety seasonal flu:

- Fever (except as otherwise noted)
- Cough
- Sore throat
- Runny or stuffy nose
- Body aches
- Headache
- Chills
- Fatigue

The CDC recommends a policy that can only be described as "an ounce of prevention is worth a pound of cure" when it comes to the flu. Get your flu shot every year and follow these steps to help you stop spreading your germs everywhere (and help you to stop picking up other people's germs):

- Stay away from sick people (you could catch what they have).
- If you're sick, stay away from healthy people (you don't want to share).
- Cover your face when you cough (this is a huge pet peeve with me—cover your cough).
- Keep your hands out of your mouth, stop picking your nose, and don't rub your eyes (now I really sound like my mom—I need to call her).
- Wash up. Mom was right; you need to wash your hands, especially if you're being good and covering your cough like you're supposed to (or being bad and picking your nose).

You may be wondering how H1N1 (the illness formerly known as *swine flu*) differs from the regular flu. Simple; it makes you sicker. Otherwise, the symptoms are the same.

PNEUMONIA

When the flu gets a little overzealous, it can result in a lung infection called *pneumonia*. Pneumonia can also come as a result of specific bacteria in the lungs.

Signs of pneumonia include:

- Coughing
- Fever
- Fatigue
- Nausea
- Vomiting
- Rapid breathing or shortness of breath
- Chills
- Chest pain

Don't treat pneumonia much more differently than you would the flu. The biggest problem with pneumonia is how it affects your breathing. Treat pneumonia by treating your shortness of breath (see Chapter 19).

COMMON COLDS

The common cold is a result of infection with a rhinovirus (which literally means *nose germs*). Rhinoviruses are pretty hardy compared to a lot of other germs. They can live up to 3 hours on surfaces, which means you can get a cold from a telephone long after the person who infected you hung up and left the room.

Even worse, you're not going to feel sick until a couple of days after you're infected. Just in case you are part of a lost race of super humans and have never had a cold, here are the symptoms:

- Sore throat
- Runny or stuffy nose
- Swollen sinuses
- Sneezing
- Coughing
- Headache
- Fatigue

There is no cure for the common cold. Personally, I'm a big fan of homemade chicken soup, but the evidence of chicken soup as a cure is pretty slim. Still, it makes you feel better. Part of the reason it makes you feel better is because fluids make you feel better. Indeed, although you can't cure a cold, you can do things to relieve the symptoms:

- Get plenty of rest
- Drink lots of fluids (and eat some broth soup)

- Treat your sore throat with throat lozenges, sprays, or gargling with salt water
- Use decongestants for sinus pressure and runny noses
- Use petroleum jelly on a raw nose
- Take Advil, aspirin, or Tylenol for a headache

There is some mounting evidence that zinc will shorten the length of a cold—if you start taking it within 24 hours of the beginning of symptoms.[8] Unfortunately, there's not much good information on how much or how often you should take it. Zinc throat lozenges might make you nauseated and the FDA says not to use zinc nasal spray because some folks have reported losing their sense of smell after using it.

Antibiotics don't cure colds; they don't even treat the symptoms. If you are uncomfortable enough to call your doctor, he or she probably won't prescribe you antibiotics unless you have some other sort of bacterial infection. Antihistamines like Benadryl can help with some of the runny noses and itchy, watery eyes.

To avoid catching a cold, or spreading one, follow these simple steps:

- Wash your hands regularly and keep them away from your face until you do. If you can't wash your hands, use alcohol-based hand sanitizer gel on them.
- Stay away from folks with colds and if you have a cold, stay away from others and don't shake hands.
- Cover your sneezes and your coughs with your elbow, not your hand (this is a big one).
- Wipe surfaces in your home, car, and office with soap and water or a disinfectant cleaner.

WEST NILE VIRUS

Before H1N1—but after avian flu—there was West Nile virus. West Nile is a virus, spread by mosquitoes, that looks much like the flu at first. The disease becomes dangerous when meningitis (inflammation of the coverings of the spinal cord and brain) or encephalitis (swelling of the brain) sets in. The good news: about 80% of all folks infected with West Nile virus will not get symptoms.[9]

Then again, maybe you're more of a 20% kind of person. According to the CDC, as many as one in five of the people who get infected could have:

- Fever
- Headache

- Body aches
- Nausea
- Vomiting
- Sometimes swollen lymph glands or a skin rash on the chest, stomach, and back

Some folks recover in a few days; others—even healthy people—can stay sick for weeks. However, this isn't the worst of it. About one in 150 people infected with West Nile will end up with even more severe symptoms—in addition to those above. These symptoms linger for a long time and some can become permanent:

- High fever
- Stiff neck
- Confusion
- Can't wake up
- Tremors or convulsions
- Weakness or paralysis
- Vision loss
- Numbness

Here's the bad news: folks over 50 are more likely to get the severe symptoms. If you are experiencing any of the symptoms listed—whether you think you were bitten by a mosquito or not—it's time to seek medical attention, either through your doctor or through the emergency department.

Your best bet is to avoid getting mosquito bites (see Chapter 26). Also, if you find any dead birds in the backyard, don't touch them with your bare hands.

MENINGITIS

The meninges are the layers of protection around the brain and spinal cord. Think of these layers as the packaging your brain comes in. Fluid flows through the layers to feed the brain and spinal cord tissue and flush waste out.

These layers can become inflamed (known as *meningitis*). There are three main infections that can cause meningitis: viruses, bacteria, and fungi. Earlier, we talked about West Nile, which is just one type of virus that can cause meningitis. Viral infections are the most common cause of meningitis. Both viral and bacterial are contagious, and bacterial meningitis can be even more dangerous than viral.[10]

The symptoms of meningitis are similar to those of severe West Nile virus. There are three symptoms that—when they show up together—are the classic signs of meningitis:

- Fever
- Severe headache
- Stiff neck

Besides those, some other symptoms often show up in meningitis. If we see these, it really seals the deal:

- Sensitivity to bright light
- Fatigue or drowsiness (maybe trouble waking up)
- Nausea and vomiting
- Lack of appetite

If you have the first three symptoms, especially if they're accompanied by anything in the second list, you need a doctor. There's not much you can do for meningitis at home, but you may be able to pass it on to others (bacterial meningitis).

If it turns out you have viral meningitis, you'll probably ride it out at home. Most folks will recover in a week or so. If it is bacterial, your doctor will prescribe antibiotics for you to take. If you have other medical conditions or a weak immune system, your doctor might want to keep you in the hospital until you get better, regardless of the type of meningitis.

SHINGLES

When I was growing up, we were always told that once you had chicken pox you were never going to get it again. Well, that's not exactly true. First, you can get chicken pox several times (my daughters share a best friend who is an unfortunate repeat customer of chicken pox). Second, for some of us, the virus that causes chicken pox (*varicella-zoster*) will return later in life to cause shingles.[11]

Shingles starts with an itching, tingling, or burning sensation that will be either on the chest, on the back, or wrapped around the rib cage

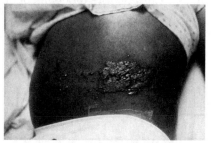

This child with shingles illustrates how the rash can wrap around one side of the torso in scaly clusters. Image courtesy of CDC

or waist. There could be a fever and maybe some weakness, but that's not always the case.

Eventually, usually within 2 or 3 days, a rash will form. You might recognize the rash; it looks just like the chicken pox bumps we got when we were kids. The biggest difference between the rash from shingles and chicken pox is that the shingles rash will only affect one side of the body, rather than the whole thing. Either the rash will cover one side of the face, or it will be a narrow band stretching around one side of the rib cage or waist from the spine to the middle of the chest.

Shingles is painful. The rash will likely scab over the same way that chicken pox does and be gone in 3 to 4 weeks, but the pain is likely to stay for much longer. Recognition is key—the faster you get in to see your doctor and get started on the proper medication, the shorter the pain should last. As soon as you see the telltale rash, make an appointment. Ideally, you want to see your doctor within 3 days of the rash appearing.

If you haven't had chicken pox in your lifetime (or the vaccine), the blisters and any drainage from them could give you chicken pox. If you've had chicken pox already, then you will probably not get them again from shingles. Like I said earlier, however, some folks are susceptible to getting chicken pox more than once. If that describes you then you should be very careful about contact with anyone who has chicken pox *or* shingles.

MRSA

There's a lot of press coverage about Methicillin-resistant *Staphylococcus aureus* (MRSA) these days. You may have heard of it. MRSA is a particularly tough form of *Staphylococcus*. *S. aureus* is a really common bug. It lives in the noses of more than one out of four people in the United States. That's a lot of bacteria.

MRSA is much less common than the garden-variety staph and much more robust. Currently, it's thought that only about 2% of folks are hosting MRSA.[12]

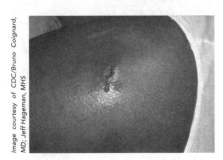

Image courtesy of CDC/Bruno Coignard, MD; Jeff Hageman, MHS

MRSA is immune to the typical antibiotics used to treat regular staph infections. Because of that, MRSA usually causes much stronger and more severe reactions, especially if it's caught in a hospital or other health care setting.

MRSA infections are often skin infections, although the bacteria can settle in other parts of the body. The typical skin infection looks like a boil or a red bump surrounded by red skin. MRSA infections are often mistaken for spider bites.[13]

The most important thing you can do for MRSA infections is to prevent them. The CDC recommends cleanliness, which is never a bad policy. Specifically:

- Regularly wash your hands. If that's not possible, use an alcohol-based hand gel.
- Cover your cuts and scratches with a bandage until they're healed.
- Don't touch other people's wounds, even if they're covered with a bandage.
- Don't share towels, toothbrushes, and razors.

FOOD POISONING

First of all, food poisoning isn't usually poisoning at all. We're really talking about food-borne illnesses. Most food-borne illnesses are caused by a few bacteria and viruses. The bacteria are *Campylobacter*, *Salmonella*, and *Escherichia coli O157:H7*. The group of viruses is the Norwalk viruses, notorious for shutting down cruise ships.[14, 15]

I could spend a whole chapter just on food-borne illnesses and all the specifics each bug brings to the table (pun intended). Instead, let's boil this down (there I go again) to the important information: how to stay safe and when to call the doctor.

Staying safe is a simple four-step process:[16]

1. *Clean:* Keep work surfaces, containers, utensils, and your hands clean while preparing and serving food. Wash everything with soap and water between uses.
2. *Separate:* Raw foods don't touch or share surfaces with cooked foods and raw meats don't touch or share surfaces with raw fruits and veggies.
3. *Cook:* Make sure whatever you cook gets to the recommended temperature in order to kill all the bugs.
4. *Chill:* Leftovers get stored and refrigerated promptly after preparation for initial meal.

There are a few symptoms common to almost every case of food poisoning: abdominal cramps, diarrhea, nausea, and vomiting. Once you get food poisoning, you're likely to recover just fine. On the other hand, call the doctor if you get any of the following:

- Fever
- Bloody stools

- Food poisoning that lasts more than 3 days
- Vomiting keeps you from keeping fluid down
- Decreased urination
- Dry mouth
- Feeling dizzy when you stand up

URINARY TRACT INFECTIONS

Urinary tract infections (UTIs) are one of the most common types of infection I see in my older patients. I call it a "silent" infection. By that I mean that plenty of folks don't know they have a UTI, even though it's affecting them.

Lots of my UTI patients call 911 for symptoms that don't scream UTI: confusion and weakness are two I see often. Once we get there and start asking questions, I realize that most folks had other, more typical symptoms; they just didn't realize they did.

CRANBERRY JUICE AND UTI

The first time I heard about the connection between cranberries and UTIs, I was a brand new paramedic, wide-eyed and gullible to all types of holistic treatments. Now I'm a grizzled old skeptic. If it was really that easy to treat things as common as UTIs with a simple food, wouldn't it be a much less common infection?

It turns out that cranberries do help prevent UTIs—a little bit, anyway.[17]

Here's the scoop: cranberries in some form, taken every day without fail, will help reduce the chance of a UTI by about 10% to 15%, especially in sexually active women who struggle with recurrent UTIs.

There's one really big problem with that (at least as far as I'm concerned): you have to drink cranberry juice. I don't like cranberry juice. Indeed, the only thing cranberry I like is my wife's homemade cranberry sauce at Thanksgiving. It's unlikely that my yearly intake of more than my fair share of brandy-laced cranberry sauce is going to shield me from the scourge of urinary bacteria. I'll take my chances sans cranberry intake for the other 364 days of the year.

So my recommendation is to drink cranberry juice if you like it (none of the studies looked at modern-day cranberry juice cocktails). If you don't have a taste for cranberry juice like me, I think you'll be fine.

The symptoms of a UTI are:

- Cloudy, dark, or bloody urine
- Foul-smelling urine
- Sometimes a fever
- Pain or burning when urinating
- Lower abdominal cramps or lower back pain
- Feels like you have to pee, even when you don't

If you notice any of these symptoms, it's worth a call to the doctor before the UTI gets worse. If it starts on a weekend, you can wait until Monday. However, be sure to call the doctor if the symptoms don't go away after 2 days.

As a UTI gets more severe, there are more severe symptoms to go with it. These are the symptoms that should prompt a visit to the ER:

- Confusion
- Fatigue or weakness
- Fever
- Flank, back, abdomen, or groin pain
- Flushed and/or hot skin
- Chills
- Cold sweats (night sweats)

The doctor is going to give you antibiotics for treatment. Be sure to take them all and to call the doctor if any symptoms of a UTI come back after treatment starts. Drink plenty of fluids to help flush out the infection. If you have a medical condition and are restricted from drinking fluids, call your doctor and ask him how much you should drink.

VOMITING AND DIARRHEA

As miserable as they are, vomiting and diarrhea have a function. When we get an infection in our stomach or intestines—called *gastroenteritis* (see Chapter 21)—our bodies either toss the bad cookies out or run them through to get rid of the bacteria. We do the same thing when we get blood or mucous in our gastrointestinal tract. When your body doesn't like it in there, it gets it out.

In most cases, you just have to ride out vomiting and diarrhea when it's related to an infection. Drink fluids when you can. If you have vomiting or diarrhea longer than 3 days, call the doctor. If you get weak or dizzy after lots of vomiting or diarrhea, call an ambulance.

ON THE INTERNET

- www.flu.gov
- www.cdc.gov/mrsa
- coldflu.about.com

IV
Surviving the Environment

24

Getting Too Hot

Quick Decisions

Are you (or the person)...
Unconscious?
Confused?
Nauseated?   YES
Too weak to stand?   to one   CALL 911
Having red and dry skin? or more
Feeling a throbbing headache?   NO?

Are you (or the person)...
Sweating?   Get out of
Able to walk?   the heat
Able to drink fluids?   YES   and drink
Able to remember: to all   sports drinks,
What you're doing?   milk, or
Where you are?   water
Who you're with?
What day it is?

As we age, we lose the ability to respond to extreme temperatures. Sometimes it's simply because of getting older, but in many cases it has to do with medical conditions or the treatments for our medical conditions.

The CDC lumps heat-related illness into something dubbed *heat stress*, which includes heat exhaustion and heatstroke. Let's take the worst one first.

HEATSTROKE

Heatstroke is the worst condition caused by heat. It occurs when heat exhaustion is left untreated and core body temperature rises to dangerously high levels. Heatstroke is a medical emergency that can lead to coma, seizures, brain damage, and death. Here are the signs and symptoms of heatstroke according to the CDC:

- High body temperature (above 103°F)
- Red, hot, and dry skin (no sweating)
- Pounding pulse
- Throbbing headache
- Dizziness
- Nausea

If you suspect someone is suffering from heatstroke, here's what to do:

1. Call 911 immediately!
2. Move the person somewhere cooler. Air conditioning is best; shade is better than nothing.
3. Strip off as much clothing as possible.
4. Put ice on the armpits, groin, and neck area to cool the person.
5. Don't give a person with heatstroke anything to drink.

161

DON'T GET SICK ON HOT DAYS

You might not be able to afford the high cost of electricity to run an air conditioner or maybe you don't even have that option. Maybe the power went out and you couldn't run the cooler if you wanted to.

Besides running a fan and spraying yourself with water to cool off, here are some steps the CDC recommends for avoiding heat stress:

- Drink a nonalcoholic glass of fluid every 15 to 20 minutes, at least one gallon each day (I don't think a full gallon is necessary for everyone; see *How Much Water is Enough?*)
- Wear light-colored, loose-fitting clothing
- When indoors without air conditioning, open windows—if outdoor air quality permits—and use fans
- Take cool showers or baths (or a dip in the pool)
- If you feel dizzy, weak, or overheated, go to a cool place. Sit or lie down, drink water, and wash your face with cool water. If you don't feel better soon, call 911.
- Work during cooler hours of the day when possible, or distribute the workload evenly throughout the day
- Look for signs of heat illness in yourself and others, especially signs of heatstroke

If the person is conscious enough to follow commands, he or she might be suffering from heat exhaustion rather than heatstroke.

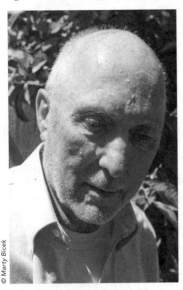

© Marty Bicek

HEAT EXHAUSTION

Heat exhaustion—like heatstroke—is also caused by increased body temperature, usually together with dehydration (fluid loss). It doesn't have to be hot for you to get heat exhaustion. Plenty of football fans have developed heat exhaustion in the stands on chilly days because they're bundled in layers of thermal undies and down jackets, especially if they're cheering hard the whole game.

Heat exhaustion can lead to heatstroke if not treated in time. Treatment might require medical intervention, but often you can take care of mild heat exhaustion without calling 911. Here are the signs and symptoms of heat exhaustion according to the CDC:

- Heavy sweating—and skin might feel cool and clammy from all that moisture
- Paleness
- Muscle cramps
- Fatigue or drowsiness
- Weakness
- Dizziness
- Headache
- Nausea or vomiting
- Fainting
- Weak, thready pulse
- Fast, shallow breathing

HOW MUCH WATER IS ENOUGH?

Many medical texts and nutrition articles advise healthy adults in comfortable temperatures with little physical activity to drink eight 8-ounce glasses of water every day. In fact, there is no scientific evidence for this advice.[18]

There's water in almost everything we eat or drink. The juice in your New York strip steak, the broth in your chicken noodle soup, and that big, cold glass of milk you use to wash your cookies down contain water. An attempt to figure out just how much water we actually take in on any given day may have accidentally led to the erroneous advice to drink water nearly constantly.

Some other conventions of medical advice concerning fluid intake are also wrong, such as telling us that caffeinated drinks and those containing alcohol don't count toward our total fluid intake. The idea is that since these substances are typically diuretics (they make you pee), drinking them leads to dehydration. That belief is a bit overblown.

The truth is that high concentrations of alcohol (liquor, wine, and sometimes even beer) can lead you to pee out more than you take in. On the other hand, a small amount of alcohol in a beverage won't discount all the fluid you get from drinking it. Caffeine becomes less of a diuretic the more often you drink it.[19]

Your best bet is to talk to your doctor about the right amount of fluids to drink, but remember: milk and other beverages count toward your total intake, and even caffeine and alcohol aren't total losses.

Much of the treatment for heat exhaustion is the same as for heatstroke, except it might not be necessary to call 911 right away. Here's what to do:

1. If the person is confused or unconscious, call 911.
2. As with heatstroke, move the person somewhere cooler. Air conditioning is best; shade is better than nothing.
3. Remove as much of the person's clothing as possible.
4. If the person is awake and talking, he or she can drink water or a sports drink like Gatorade.

Just like anything else in medical care, heat illnesses aren't either/or. In other words, it's not like the body chugs along just fine until heat exhaustion suddenly starts, then switches to heatstroke after a few minutes. It happens gradually, so you may recognize signs from both lists (the person is red and hot, but still sweating, for example).

The key is to seek medical attention when you feel overwhelmed. As we've already seen, a good rule of thumb is to call 911 whenever the brain starts to malfunction, either through confusion or unconsciousness.

A NOTE ABOUT MEDICATIONS

Medications that control blood pressure or heart arrhythmias are especially hard on the body's ability to control temperature or can lead to dehydration. Some antibiotics and other classes of medications can make your skin much more susceptible to the sun.

It's important to be aware of how you're feeling, especially in extreme temperatures or when you're exerting an unusual amount of physical activity. Don't ever stop or adjust your medication for fear of dehydration or sun exposure. Instead, call your doctor and explain your concerns. Your doctor might be able to prescribe a different option or suggest things you could do differently.

Your pharmacist could also make suggestions on how to stay cool or hydrated when taking certain medications.

DEHYDRATION

Dehydration doesn't have to be from heat stress. In fact, most instances of dehydration in seniors don't have anything to do with heat.

Sweating from being too hot surely leads to dehydration, but so can certain medications (blood pressure and heart medications especially) and infections. Simply not drinking enough water is also a common cause of dehydration. It's important to stay adequately hydrated, but the most common recommendation for drinking water is a little bit of a myth.

The important thing with dehydration is to recognize it. Be aware of your own body. Look for the signs and symptoms of dehydration, especially if you're really hot or really sick:

- Dizziness
- Headache
- Nausea and vomiting
- Weakness
- Dry mouth and nose
- Inability to urinate

The more severe the dehydration, the more likely you will need to call 911. Like heat illness, dehydration comes on gradually, so listen to your body. Don't be afraid to call 911 if you get dizzy or weak.

On the Internet

- emergency.cdc.gov/disasters/extremeheat
- www.weather.gov/om/heat/index.shtml

25

Getting Too Cold

Quick Decisions

Are you (or the person)...
Unconscious?
Confused?
Too weak to stand?
Uncoordinated?
Too cold to think?
Numb in fingers or toes?

YES to one or more ➤ **CALL 911**

NO ➤ Get out of the cold, bundle up, pour some hot cocoa, and read on

Do you get cold more easily than you used to? Studies show that you don't react to cold temperatures at 65 the same way you did when you were 25. When we're cold, we're supposed to divert our blood away from our skin so it stays deep inside and heat can't escape.

Getting too cold is a serious concern, especially for seniors living alone and on a fixed income. If you're trying to conserve on the heating bill, make sure you're warm enough and have plenty to eat. Staying warm burns calories, so you want to be sure the pantry is well-stocked if the heat is going to be turned down.

Getting too cold is known as *hypothermia*, and hypothermia is a bad place to be. Our bodies produce heat naturally, all day long. The way it's supposed to work is that we produce heat from within and some of that heat is released through our skin and through our breath out into the world around us. We have the ability, through how much blood is allowed to flow near the surface of the skin, to regulate how much heat is lost.

Hypothermia is like losing the race. Your body is unable to produce as much heat as it is losing. As we get older, our bodies don't burn calories as fast, which means we don't make as much heat. Plus, our ability to react to cold weather is impaired as we age. Altogether, we don't make as much heat and we lose more of it to the environment, making us susceptible to hypothermia.

Normal body temperature is about 98.6°F (37°C). When your temperature drops below 95°F (35°C), you are suffering from hypothermia. By the time we are suffering from hypothermia, we're already behind the curve. Our bodies are now losing heat faster than they can make more.

The first sign of hypothermia is shivering. Your body reacts to the loss of heat by trying to make more. Shivering only works for a few minutes. Your body will continue to shiver only as long as you have enough energy to do that. Once you get cold enough, the shivering will stop, but don't take that as a sign that you're getting better. Shivering is only one sign of hypothermia; see the sidebar *Recognizing Hypothermia* for more.

167

RECOGNIZING HYPOTHERMIA

Normal body temperature is around 98.6°F (37°C). It can be a little higher or a little lower, but not too much.

When your temperature drops below 95°F (35°C), you are suffering from hypothermia. The symptoms of hypothermia aren't obvious when they are happening to us, so it's important to pay attention when you're in the cold and definitely keep an eye on others who are in the cold with you.

- Shivering or chills
- Exhaustion
- Confusion
- Fumbling fingers
- Memory loss (can't concentrate)

As hypothermia gets worse, it gets even harder to recognize the symptoms in yourself. If you think someone else has hypothermia, you need to call 911 if they start falling asleep and can't wake up or have slurred speech.

Fixing hypothermia is simple: get warm. There is a trick to it, however. We lose heat through skin all over our bodies, but there are certain areas more prone to heat loss: soles of the feet, palms of the hands, the neck, face, and head. When you bundle up to try to get warm, be sure to cover those areas as well. Letting your head and hands get cold while you're trying to warm up your chest and belly will slow you down.

WHY DO WE SHIVER?

You finish watching the spring musical revue at your grandchild's school and stand in the parking lot talking to family for 20 minutes. It's a brisk night and you feel yourself getting chilly. Pretty soon you're shivering.

Our bodies work like cars. We burn fuel (cars burn gas; we burn top sirloin and sweet potatoes) and from that fuel we get heat and energy. Usually, heat is a byproduct of us burning calories for the energy to move and think. When we're too cold (*hypothermic*), we burn calories to stay warm and energy is the byproduct.

That excess energy has to go somewhere. It doesn't just float away into the air. So, to use up the energy we make while we're burning Brussels sprouts for heat, our muscles get excited and start shivering.

If you suspect hypothermia is causing someone (even yourself) to be confused or have slurred speech, call 911 immediately. Once hypothermia gets bad enough to affect the brain, it's very difficult to warm up without medical intervention.

In really severe cases of hypothermia, the heart slows and blood pressure drops so low that the person may appear dead. Often, people with such severe hypothermia can be revived. It's important to call 911 and start CPR on any person of suspected hypothermia who isn't breathing, even if you think it's too late.

FROSTBITE

It doesn't take very low temperatures to lead to hypothermia; leaving the heat off on a cold night will do the trick. Frostbite, on the other hand, requires freezing temperatures, but you don't have to be outside.

THAWING FROSTBITE

To thaw frostbitten tissues:

1. Protect the person from the freezing temperatures.
2. Remember: don't thaw frostbitten tissues if it is possible they could freeze again.
3. Cover the frostbitten body part in water that is about 98 to 105°F (36.7° to 40.5°C; a little warmer than normal body temperature)
4. When the water cools, add more. Keep the water temperature as consistent as possible.

As soon as you can, get medical care even if the frostbite is already thawed.

Frostbite is frozen skin and muscle tissue. Sometimes it's called freezer burn or a cold burn, which makes a lot of sense when you see it. Frostbite looks a lot like a burn and the damage to skin is quite similar. How well and how quickly frostbite heals depends—like a burn—on how deep the damage goes.

Frostbite is most common on the parts of the body furthest from

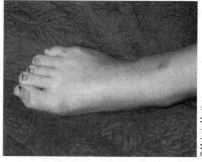

© Melanie Martinez

the heart, where blood flow isn't as robust: nose, earlobes, fingers, and toes are the most common. Usually, exposure is the key. When those low-blood-flow areas are exposed to freezing temperatures for too long (the colder the temperature, the less time it takes), the skin and muscle tissues will begin to freeze.

WILL BRANDY WARM ME UP?

When I was growing up, television cartoons always portrayed St. Bernard dogs running through the snow with casks of brandy slung around their necks. Presumably, this brandy was going to save lost souls trapped in the Swiss Alps. (Ever notice how much drinking and carousing went on in those Saturday cartoons?)

As it turns out, those St. Bernards were actually carrying mail, not brandy. The cartoons were perpetuating a myth about the benefits of drinking alcohol to warm you up when you're feeling a bit chilly.

Drinking alcohol makes you feel flushed because it shifts blood to the skin. The skin feels the warm blood soaking into it and we get that warm, fuzzy glow.

What your skin doesn't feel is all the heat that it loses to the outside environment when your blood rushes to the surface.

Thanks to that brandy, we're actually getting colder, not warmer.

Alcohol doesn't warm you up and is a surefire way to suffer from hypothermia when you're exposed to the cold.

Frostbite doesn't always come from outside exposure to cold temperatures; sometimes we do it to ourselves. It's possible to get frostbite from icing an injury (see Chapter 16). My own daughter suffered frostbite from keeping ice on her injured leg too long.

If you're concerned about frostbite (for instance, you've been climbing Mt. Hood and are wondering about the loss of feeling in your feet) look for these signs:

- Redness and swelling (similar to a burn)
- Blisters
- White or waxy appearance to the skin
- Numbness or tingling
- Extreme pain
- Inability to move injured areas

Treatment for frostbite depends on whether you have access to medical care. If so, call 911 or go to the emergency department for immediate care. If not, you can thaw frostbitten tissues yourself, but you have to follow one simple rule: don't let the damaged tissues freeze again. If you're likely to still be exposed to freezing temperatures, it's better *not* to thaw frostbite.

ON THE INTERNET

• www.bt.cdc.gov/disasters/winter/guide.asp

26

Spiders, Snakes, and Other Critters

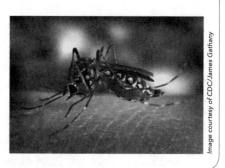

Image courtesy of CDC/James Gathany

A nimal bites—dogs, cats, platypuses, orangutans, dolphins, and humans—are covered in Chapter 17 (puncture wounds). Basically, they're just puncture wounds that need to be cleaned really well. Watch them carefully for infection. Besides mammals, there are lots of other things that can bite or sting, like spiders, snakes, and insects.

Bug bites are bug bites. Sometimes we assume they are spiders. Sometimes we know they're mosquitoes or chiggers. Sometimes we find a scorpion or a centipede. Most of the time, however, we don't see anything other than a red mark that we figure must have come from some critter or another.

I'll let you in on a secret: Most little red marks aren't from critters at all. Most of the time, they're skin infections like *staphylococcus* or *streptococcus*. Some folks believe that a bite by some miniature critter might be why these skin infections take hold in the first place, but either way they're still skin infections.

That's not to say there aren't really biting spiders lurking about; black widows certainly have a nasty bite. We know that chiggers, bed bugs, and mosquitoes will feast upon us if we let them. So let's take a look at some of the known biting (and stinging) bugs, including spiders.

Creepy Crawly Critters

There aren't statistics available for which bugs bite the most, but I think it's safe to say mosquitoes and ticks would be near the top of the list. Both of these bugs really don't like DEET, a form of insect repellant. Using DEET when you're outside can help protect you from mosquitoes, ticks, and other biting insects.

That's important, because while itching from a mosquito bite might seem like nothing more than an annoyance, they carry dangerous viruses.

Mosquito Bites

Mosquito bites are the epitome of an ounce of prevention being worth a pound of cure. There's not much you can do for mosquito bites once you get them. Some very lucky people do not react to mosquito bites, but the rest of us mortals will itch. The itching is because we are mildly allergic to the mosquito's saliva.

To fix the itching, creams are your best bet. Calamine lotion and Benadryl cream help with the itching. You can also find lotions with both calamine and Benadryl combined. Insect-sting swabs can be used directly on the bites to numb them.

Scratching mosquito bites can damage the skin and open them up to infection, but the real danger of mosquito bites comes from the viruses they carry. West Nile virus, malaria, Yellow fever, Dengue fever, and several other illnesses can all be transmitted by a mosquito bite.

The most important thing to remember about mosquitoes is to let your doctor know if you have any flu-like symptoms after being bitten. Many of the viruses mosquitoes carry look very much like the flu at first.

To protect yourself from mosquitoes, the CDC offers these tips:

- Stay indoors at dawn and dusk when mosquitoes are the most active (I know that's tough—those are my favorite times of the day)
- Use window screens to keep mosquitoes outside
- Wear long sleeves
- Use insect repellant with DEET, picaridin, or oil of lemon eucalyptus (DEET is the best, so unless you're really against chemicals, I recommend it)
- Get rid of standing water in the yard (other than a well-kept swimming pool); mosquitoes breed in standing water

Tick Bites

Like mosquitoes, ticks are bearers of bad news. Not only that, but ticks are extra gross. They bury their heads under the skin when they bite and they spread viruses that cause—among other things—Lyme disease and Rocky Mountain spotted fever. It's important to let your doctor know if you were bitten by a tick and experience the following symptoms:

- Fever
- Headache

- Stiff neck
- Body aches
- Fatigue

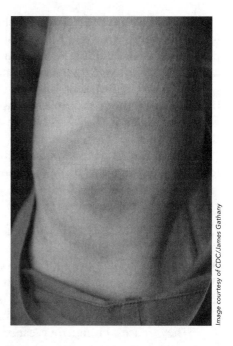

Image courtesy of CDC/James Gathany

If these symptoms are seen, even several days later, seek medical help immediately.

Plus, Lyme disease often has a skin rash. In many cases, the rash looks like a bull's-eye pattern with concentric circles of red and white.

When a tick has buried her head under the skin (it's almost always the female), you will need to remove it carefully. There are all sorts of home remedies for removing ticks, from burning them off to smothering them in petroleum jelly. Home tick remedies often don't work and in some cases can actually lead to worsening infection. In reality, there's only one safe method: pulling them out with tweezers.

To remove a tick, follow these steps from the CDC:

1. Grasp the tick with tweezers as close to the skin as possible.
2. Pull the tick straight out with gentle, constant pressure. If you pull too hard, you might tear the tick apart and leave some behind.
3. Make sure all of the tick was removed, including all of the tick's mouthparts.
4. If any part of the tick is missing, seek medical attention immediately.
5. Don't touch the tick with bare hands and save it in an airtight container.

If you're in an area where ticks live, keep an eye on the warm, moist parts of your body for ticks: armpits, groin, neck, back of the knees, and behind your ears.

CHIGGERS

Chiggers are baby mites, which are related to ticks. They bite in a similar way, but their mouthparts are smaller and they don't bury their heads. Chiggers inject saliva to liquefy skin cells and suck the liquid out. Most of us react to the saliva with intense itching.

Chiggers hate DEET, so use that bug spray if you're in an area known for chiggers. They love warm, moist places and go for the ankles. You'll probably feel the itching before you notice the chiggers. Once you have chiggers, you'll have to actively get them off.

Take a bath. Lather up the area with soap, rinse and repeat. They'll be hard to see, so lather and rinse a couple of times to get them all.

If a bath isn't possible, rub them off with a clean towel or cloth. Follow that up with a bath when you can.

The itching is a curse you will have to wait out. It may take as long as 10 to 14 days for the itching to stop. Calamine and Benadryl lotions might help.

DON'T LET THE BED BUGS BITE

Bed bugs are like disco and mullets; they're making a comeback, even though nobody really wants them. Bed bugs are just that: bugs that like to live in beds. Bed bugs, like ticks and mosquitoes, feed on the blood of people and animals. They like to feed while we sleep.

They cause itching (they cause me to itch just writing this). If you scratch them too much, you can get a skin infection like staph or strep, but bed bugs don't spread any known diseases.

They're ugly. They stink. They ruin your mattress. However, they're not dangerous.

BEE STINGS

Bee stings hurt like the dickens and can be very dangerous if you're allergic to bee venom. The venom of bees, wasps, and hornets reacts the same regardless of which insect stings you. Some bees have a barb on the end of the stinger that holds it in place after the sting. Those bee stingers have a little sac of venom that keeps pumping after the bee has stung you and flown away.

It's important to get bee stingers out as quickly as possible. The oldest myth in first aid is the one about scraping off bee stingers. It's much more important to get the stinger out quickly. Most of the time, you can just brush the stinger away. They're tiny and it doesn't take much to knock them off. If the stinger doesn't come out by brushing it off, pick it off with your fingers.

If you're allergic to bee stings, you need to react quickly (see *Anaphylaxis* and *How to Use an EpiPen* in Chapter 19 for more information).

SPIDER BITES

There's a tendency to blame spiders for any swollen, red blister or lesion on the skin that we can't explain. In fact, research has repeatedly shown that unexplained sores on the skin are more likely to be skin infections than spider bites.[20] Spiders aren't even to blame for causing the infections.[21]

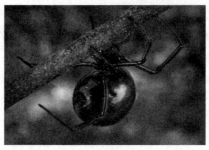

Black widow spider; Image courtesy of CDC/James Gathany

Most spiders are venomous. They need to be venomous to hunt. However, most spiders are too small and their venom is too weak to be dangerous to us.

In the United States there are only three spiders that are known to cause serious reactions: black widow, brown recluse, and the hobo spider. The worst is the black widow spider. Black widows have venom that's toxic to the nervous system. Black widow bites are almost never fatal but they can be very painful. Call your doctor or go to the hospital if you get bitten by a black widow and start feeling cramps or pain in your abdomen, back, or thighs.

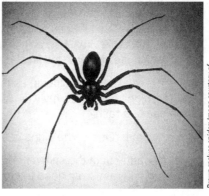

Brown recluse spider; Image courtesy of CDC/Andrew J. Brooks

Brown recluse spiders can cause very nasty reactions, even leading to loss of muscle tissue. However, the bite of the brown recluse is extremely rare. In fact, these guys are called *recluses* for a reason: they don't like to come in contact with people.

Hobo spider bites cause very similar reactions to brown recluse bites. Even though hobo spiders only live in the Pacific Northwest and brown recluse spiders only live in the southeast United States, patients and doctors will often attribute reactions to the wrong type of spider.

Many of the sores blamed on brown recluses and hobo spiders are really skin infections, which makes diagnosing them difficult. Spiders are notoriously difficult to identify, even if you have a specimen to examine. You'll have to talk to a doctor if you think you've been bitten by a brown recluse or hobo spider.

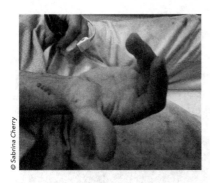

© Sabrina Cherry

SNAKE BITES

There are two types of venomous snakes in the United States: pit vipers and coral snakes. Rattlesnakes—of the pit viper family—far outnumber any other species of venomous snake around. If you're going to have the misfortune of getting bitten by a snake, chances are it'll be a rattler.

First thing I want to say is: no cutting and sucking. The old snake bite kits used to come with a razor blade or scalpel and some sort of extraction contraption to suck out the poison. Sucking out the venom doesn't work.

WEST NILE HITS HOME

In the summer of 2005, West Nile virus was a big problem in my hometown. The newspaper ran weekly statistics and updates of victims, and neighbors had been finding dead birds in their yards. My wife, Melanie, and I sat in the backyard on a warm August evening. Suddenly, she slapped her leg.

The mosquito was killed in the act of biting, and we joked about how Mel was going to get West Nile now. A few days later she started complaining of body aches and a fever, so again I teased her about getting West Nile virus. I did a little research on the symptoms of West Nile, which are similar to the flu and exactly what she was experiencing.

About a week into her illness, as the flu-like symptoms just hung on and wouldn't get better, my wife yelled from the shower, "Does West Nile cause a rash?"

"Yes," I said. "One of the signs is a rash."

Mel stepped out of the shower and said, "Like this?" She was covered in a rash from head to toe.

Mel did indeed have West Nile and developed the rash along with mild cases of encephalitis and meningitis. We hadn't used bug spray in our backyard that night because mosquitoes had always been nothing more than an annoyance. It shows just how dangerous a little mosquito can be.

The only thing that will really help you in the case of a snake bite is a hospital. You'll need to get help fast and get to the emergency department where they can give you the antivenin. In the meantime, or if getting you to the hospital is going to take a while, you can wrap the arm or leg with a compression bandage to slow the venom's march toward the heart.

I can't stress this enough, however. *The most important thing you need is a hospital.* Call 911 and get to the ER pronto.

MARINE BITES AND STINGS

Sea anemones and jellyfish cause the most stings at the beach, although you're more likely to suffer from sunburn than a jellyfish sting. The American Heart Association (AHA) just added jellyfish sting treatment to its first aid guidelines in 2010. They recommend the following:

- Pull off any remaining tentacles with a stick or other object—just don't use your bare hands or you'll get another sting.
- Rinse with hot water. There's a recommended temperature, but more importantly the AHA recommends rinsing with water as hot as you can comfortably stand it.
- After 10 minutes or when you run out of hot water, rinse with plain distilled white vinegar.

I want to point out that *nowhere* in the AHA recommendations does it say to urinate on the jellyfish sting. Despite what you may have heard to the contrary, peeing on a jellyfish sting is not a treatment—it's just gross.

Lastly, I'd like to address stingrays, because they have gotten a few lucky shots in the last few years and folks are now quite afraid of them. Stingrays sting pretty often and while their barbed stingers hurt terribly, they are rarely fatal. Treat the barbed stinger that's still stuck in the skin as an impaled object (see Chapter 17).

ON THE INTERNET

- www.cdc.gov
- firstaid.about.com/od/bitesstings

27
Poisons and Poisonings

There are a lot of different things that can poison you in your own home. I could never cover all of them in this little chapter; that would require a whole other book.

Fortunately, there aren't too many different ways of handling poisonings, at least for the layperson. For the most part, it doesn't matter what the poison is; Poison Control can guide you in how to respond. Keep the phone number handy. Post it anywhere that poisonings might happen (garage, storage shed, bathroom, and mudroom are common places) and also next to the main phone in the house.

The Poison Control National telephone number is 1-800-222-1222. If you think you've been poisoned (or someone else has) don't panic. Follow these tips from the American Association of Poison Control Centers (AAPCC):[22]

- For any person who is unconscious or not responding, call 911, whether you think it's from exposure to poison or not.
- For poison in the eyes, flush both eyes with plain tap water (even if the poison only got into one) for at least 15 to 20 minutes. Call Poison Control.
- For a small amount of poison on the skin, rinse it off with lots of water for at least 20 minutes. Call Poison Control.
- For a small amount of poison on clothing, remove the clothing then rinse with running water all over the potentially contaminated body areas for at least 20 minutes. Call Poison Control.
- For large amounts of poison on the skin or clothes, call 911 immediately.
- For inhaled poisons, move to fresh air, preferably outside. Call Poison Control.

If you take too much medication or the wrong drugs (such as your spouse's), call Poison Control.

NOT EVERY POISON HAS A SKULL AND CROSSBONES ON THE LABEL

Before you could buy it over the counter, lice shampoo was only available by prescription. It came in the same type of bottle as cough medicine and liquid antibiotics (my daughter always asked for liquid amoxicillin, "the pink medicine," whenever she had an earache). Lice shampoo was indistinguishable from any other prescription liquid except for the label.

Years ago I responded in the ambulance to a man who, intending to treat his cough, took a swig from a bottle of lice shampoo. I don't condone his dosing methods because you should never drink cough medicine or any other medication straight from the bottle, but in this case it was worse. He certainly wasn't drinking what he thought he was drinking.

When we arrived at his house, he was waiting for us at the sidewalk by his front lawn. He didn't appear to be in any distress and he said he felt fine. After the man realized he had drunk from the wrong bottle—first by the hideous taste then by finally reading the label—he called Poison Control. They told him to call 911 immediately.

We put him right into the ambulance and drove him to the hospital less than 5 minutes away. Before we got to the ER he started vomiting, his eyes were watering, and he became incontinent. Minutes after putting him in the emergency bed he started having seizures.

The man survived, but not because of anything we did. Lice shampoo serves a purpose, and it is also a deadly poison. Being around pesticides all my life, I assumed that anything really dangerous would not be placed in the hands of just anyone or at least have a label expressing how toxic it is. The man was lucky he lived so close to the hospital. After that, I've made an effort to call Poison Control myself if I'm unfamiliar with the potential poison.

If you swallow something that isn't supposed to be swallowed, drink a small amount of milk or water and call Poison Control.

A note about calling 911 for a poisoning: In most parts of the country, the 911 center will connect you to a Poison Control center even as they are sending you an ambulance. Never hesitate to call 911 if you think it's an emergency. In some cases, Poison Control operators will let the 911 center know whether to continue the ambulance or not.

PESTICIDES

When I was growing up, I lived on a dairy farm. We had all kinds of ethyl-methyl bad stuff piled up in every corner of the barn and the shop. It was everywhere and I was completely oblivious to how dangerous some of these toxins really were.

Pesticides were probably the worst of these poisons and that's true of your home as well. There are two very common pesticides you're likely to run into around the house: rat poison (*rodenticide*) and bug spray (*insecticide*). Each works in its own way.

Rat poison is related to Coumadin, a common blood thinner. Indeed, some rat poisons actually list warfarin, a generic form of Coumadin, on the label. The idea with rat poison is that the rat gets such thin blood that it develops massive bleeding and simply runs out of blood.

Not surprisingly, that's what happens to humans when they ingest rat poison as well. If there's any possibility that rat poison has been ingested by a person (you or someone else), it's time to call 911.

Likewise, if insecticide is ingested or even if there's a serious exposure to copious amounts of insecticide, it's time to call 911. Insecticide is like nerve gas for bugs and it causes serious reactions to humans as well:[23]

- Headache
- Tears in the eyes
- Runny nose
- Increased saliva
- Vomiting
- Diarrhea
- Sweating
- General weakness
- Muscle twitching
- Seizures
- Shallow breathing
- Not breathing
- Dizziness
- Constricted pupils
- Abdominal pain or cramps
- Fatigue

A person having a toxic reaction to insecticide and showing these signs is in danger of having an extremely low blood pressure, slow pulse, and of course, death. If you see two or three of these symptoms show up at the same time, especially if you suspect the person may have been exposed to a poison, call 911.

BLEACH AND AMMONIA

Never mix cleaning materials. Bleach and ammonia are two very common cleaning agents that are found in many different products. Bleach and ammonia do not play well together. Mixing them creates a toxic gas that can overwhelm you, leaving you unconscious and eventually dead.

If you discover someone in a room lying on the floor unconscious next to a mop bucket, it's not a bad idea to assume he or she may have become overwhelmed by the fumes. It's really important to move the person to fresh air, but you must be careful: you could become overwhelmed as well.

Open doors and windows to start ventilating the room before trying to move the person. If the person is too big for you to move him or her quickly and easily out of the room, call 911. Breathing those same toxic fumes, especially while exerting yourself trying to move another person, is just going to result in you passing out as well. It's much better not to have a second victim and besides, if you pass out, who's going to call 911?

CARBON MONOXIDE POISONING

Carbon monoxide is a byproduct of burning things. It's in smoke from fires and exhaust from gas- or diesel-powered motors. Even though carbon monoxide is often hidden in stinky smoke and exhaust, by itself it's odorless and colorless. Carbon monoxide is a silent killer.

Red blood cells are the part of the blood that makes it red and the part that carries oxygen. Red blood cells like carbon monoxide much more than they like oxygen, so much so that red blood cells will actually let go of oxygen in order to attach to carbon monoxide. The problem is that carbon monoxide doesn't do anything for the body. We can't live on carbon monoxide.

More than 400 people in the United States die from carbon monoxide poisoning every year. There are more than 20,000 visits to the ER and over 4,000 of those have to be kept overnight (or longer) in the hospital. Deaths from carbon monoxide poisonings are most common in folks 65 and older.[24]

The problem with carbon monoxide is that we don't know when we're breathing it (since we can't smell it) and the symptoms can look just like an infection. You can be inhaling a little bit of carbon monoxide for a long time and have symptoms or get sick very quickly from inhaling a lot of carbon monoxide in a short period.

The symptoms of carbon monoxide poisoning include:

- Headache
- Nausea and vomiting
- Dizziness
- Weakness or fatigue
- Unstable gait (stumbling around)
- Confusion
- Unconscious and unable to wake up

Since multiple folks can breathe carbon monoxide fumes at the same time, people often mistake the symptoms as food poisoning or the flu. They might think they all got the infection or the food poisoning at the same time when in reality it's because they're all breathing the same air.

You may read or hear that carbon monoxide poisoning victims get very red. It does happen, but it's a very late sign. By the time someone gets very red skin from carbon monoxide poisoning, they're usually unconscious and very, very sick. Don't rely on red coloring of the skin to tell you that the problem is carbon monoxide poisoning.

Indeed, the only way to tell for sure is to keep a carbon monoxide detector in the home. Unlike smoke detectors, carbon monoxide detectors don't sound an alarm just because they detect a trace amount of carbon monoxide. Instead, if the carbon monoxide levels are really high or if a small amount of the fumes have been around for quite a while, the detector will sound an alarm.

If you have a carbon monoxide alarm and it starts beeping, go outside to the fresh air and call 911. Most fire departments have a device that allows them to check the air for carbon monoxide levels.

There are some things you can do to avoid releasing carbon monoxide fumes into your home:

- Always make sure your gas stove or oven is turned off at night. If you have a pilot light, make sure it's on and blue, not yellow.
- All gas appliances in the home (gas cooking appliances, fireplaces, water heaters, and clothes dryers) need to be properly ventilated to the outside.
- Make sure wood stoves and fireplaces are drafting smoke up the chimney properly and that the chimney is clean. Make sure the flue is open when lit.
- Never cook on an outdoor grill (gas or charcoal) indoors or under an enclosed patio.
- Never run a generator or any other gasoline- or diesel-powered motor indoors.

- Avoid using gas or oil space heaters.
- Never run a car or motorcycle engine in a garage, even if you have the door open.

On the Internet

- www.aapcc.org
- firstaid.about.com/od/poisons

28

Twisters, Earthquakes, and Other Bad Days

Not Ready Yet

If you have been told to evacuate immediately: grab your keys, get in the car and go, and read this book later.

If officials say you have time, read *What to Do If You Didn't Prepare* in this chapter.

N ot every emergency is a little emergency. Some of them are real monsters.

I grew up in a pretty mild part of California. We hardly ever saw a thunderstorm. It snowed once when I was in kindergarten and the earthquakes were always just over the hill in someone else's backyard. Our most dangerous weather phenomenon was fog (serious, white-out, can't-see-your-mailbox kind of fog, but come on, it's still just fog).

Despite our mild weather and lack of temblors, we did experience the occasional blackout. Unfortunately for us, power failures had a tendency to come in the middle of summertime. While we hardly ever saw a serious storm, we had triple-digit temperatures every year. Losing your air conditioning when it's 98°F in the shade is a life-threatening proposition for some people.

Even in our relatively mild part of foggy, hot paradise, we had to plan for the occasional bad day. Regardless of where you live and how safe you feel, disasters can affect you. Even if you don't live in tornado, hurricane, or earthquake country, you could lose power or water at any time. Plus, as we all learned the hard way on September 11, 2001, some disasters are man-made.

THE BASIC NEEDS

Whether you're planning for a hurricane, forest fire, global warming, or an invasion of space aliens, there are a few things you ought to have on hand in case regular services aren't available.

Every person has three basic necessities in this order:

1. Water
2. Food
3. Shelter and warmth

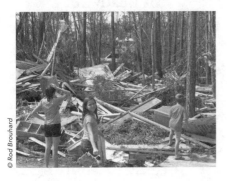

© Rod Brouhard

We can last longer without shelter (and to a lesser extent, warmth) than without food, and longer without food than without water. There are two different kinds of disasters to prepare for: the kind that requires evacuation and the kind that lets you stay home. In both cases, you'll probably have to fend for yourself for a while.

If you don't have to leave the house, then shelter is not an issue. Once you leave, however, shelter will depend on how severe the weather is. If it's really wet, cold, or hot, you're going to want to find a place to get out of the elements fairly quickly.

STOCKING THE SHELVES

In a disaster, food and water supplies will be your problem, at least for a while. Authorities at the Federal Emergency Management Agency (FEMA) recommend at least a 3-day supply of food and water, 7 days if you really want to be prepared.

Deciding how to store supplies depends on how you expect to use them. In hurricane country, you're likely to evacuate in the event of a big storm. If that's the case, stock your supplies in portable containers that are easy to load in the car. In earthquake country, there's no warning when temblors hit.

So pack your supplies to match your area. If you'll be evacuating, create an "emergency evacuation kit" that you can load in the car in 10 minutes or less. If evacuation isn't likely and you'll be stuck at home without water and power, you can simply dedicate a few shelves to emergency supplies.

It's a lot of stuff to store and a lot of stuff to carry, especially if you're not as spry and strong as you used to be. The best way to prepare is to have someone help you organize your supplies in a way that you'll be able to access them as needed in case of an emergency.

For example, you'll want to store things so you don't have to lift any heavy boxes in order to transport or access supplies. Keep water in one area and make sure the bottles aren't too heavy to lift and pour. Those big square bottles with the pour spout on the bottom would be perfect for water storage.

EMERGENCY WATER SUPPLY

Water storage recommendations are based on the myth that we need to drink 64 ounces (half a gallon) of water per person every day, but that's not really true (see *How Much Water is Enough?* in Chapter 24). Still, it's a good idea to have that water on hand in case of a true disaster. Each person in the house (and pet) should have a gallon of water per day—half to drink and the other half to use for brushing teeth, cooking, washing, and so on.

If you will be evacuating—or staying in place without power and running water—and the weather is expected to be hot, store extra water. In extremely hot temperatures it's difficult to cool off and dehydration becomes a real concern.

The FDA says bottled water (the kind you buy at the store) has a virtually unlimited shelf life. As long as the bottles aren't damaged or opened, you should be able to store your emergency water supply for a very long time.

If you use bottled water at home all the time, rotate your stock. Use the bottles you packed for an emergency and put new bottles there. That way, all your supplies will be fresh.

EMERGENCY FOOD SUPPLY

If it's in your refrigerator, it doesn't count as an emergency supply. If it can last on a shelf for a long time, you're good. Stick with food that's low sodium so you won't need to drink extra water (it's hard to find canned and long shelf-life items that aren't full of salt).

Stick with ready-to-eat items. Rice and beans have a long shelf life, but they require cooking and water to prepare. Instead, buy canned goods. You'll lose some shelf life, but you'll gain the ability to actually eat it no matter how bad the situation gets.

Plan on 2,000 calories a day per person and don't forget pet food if you have a pet. If you are regularly consuming more than 2,000 calories, then pack to keep up on your daily intake.

When I went to the Gulf Coast to help out with hurricanes Katrina and Ike, we lived on cans of beans, crackers, Pop-Tarts, beef jerky, nuts, Twinkies, and peanut butter. It's not a healthy diet, but it provided more than enough calories. At base camp we had prepared food, but when we were out in the field overnight it was all about the packages of processed goodness.

One other menu item we had plenty of was cases of military Meals Ready to Eat (MRE). When my oldest son was little, he thought these things were delicious—now that he's in the Army, he's changed his mind.

MREs are bland and—in my opinion—kind of metallic-tasting. However, they have very long shelf lives and, if you get the right kind, can provide a hot meal even without gas or electricity. Most MRE packets are at least 2,000 calories, so you'll only need to pack one per person, per day.

The MREs that provide a hot meal use a heater that is activated by putting water in a pouch. The heaters get hot enough to burn—especially if you touch it too long. Use this kind of MRE very carefully, because if you can't get food, you probably can't get medical care very easily, either.

If you're not using MREs—which nobody would eat on purpose if almost anything else was available—rotate your food the same way you rotate your water. If you have a hankering for Pop-Tarts, take them out of the emergency supplies and put the new package from the store back on the shelf. It keeps food fresh and keeps it from spoiling or expiring.

EMERGENCY SHELTER

Shelter is important for long-term evacuations. If evacuation isn't necessary, then shelter is easy—your home. On the other hand, if you have to leave, then you want to make sure you have adequate shelter for everyone going with you.

Shelter is more than a tent or a car to stay out of the elements. It also means bedding and clothing for each person (and pet, if necessary) who has to evacuate.

Adequate shelter means having insulation for the weather. If it's extremely hot outside (it gets to triple digits where I grew up), then you'll need a way to cool off. In extreme cold temperatures, make sure there are enough layers to be warm.

Sleeping bags are better than blankets for warmth, but if you have trouble getting in and out of a sleeping bag, then blankets work. If you use blankets, make sure you have enough to do the trick.

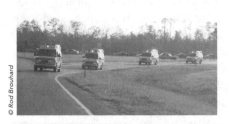

© Rod Brouhard

MAKING AN EMERGENCY EVACUATION KIT

Making a kit is all about portability and rapid deployment. It's not enough to simply have all the supplies dotted around the house. You need to make sure you can find what you need when you need it. Here are some tips for packing a useful kit:

- Store water where it won't freeze, food where it won't spoil, and everything else in an easy-to-access area.
- Pack the entire kit in small, light plastic storage boxes to make it easy to load into the car on short notice.
- Keep the food in a separate container from everything else. Bottled water can be stored and loaded separately.
- Do a dry run: pack the car ahead of time to see if it all fits and how hard it is to pack.
- Replace water once a year to maintain fresh taste. The FDA says it doesn't really expire, but that doesn't mean it won't taste like plastic after a while.

Once you've created an evacuation kit with food and any over-the-counter medications (we'll tackle prescriptions later in the chapter), write down the earliest expiration date for either food or medication. Mark the date of the earliest expiration on your calendar. On that date, replace any food or drugs that will expire in the next 6 months. Mark the next earliest date on your calendar and do it all over again on that date.

Here are recommended food and water supplies:

- Three gallons of water for each person and pet using the kit
- Three days' worth of food per person using the kit (6,000-7,500 calories per person)
- Three days' worth of pet food
- Disposable utensils, plates, and bowls (washing wastes water)
- Manual can opener
- Sharp knife
- Small cutting board
- Salt, pepper, sugar, and other spices
- Aluminum foil and plastic wrap
- Resealable plastic bags

Food and water aren't all you need if you have to evacuate. You'll also need supplies for health and hygiene, special medical conditions, clothing, shelter, light, and communication with the outside world (at least a way to hear news).

Special needs for medical conditions:

- Walkers or wheelchairs
- Hearing aid batteries (to keep them fresh, use the batteries in the kit and put new ones in whenever you need to change)

- Special foods (gluten free, sugar free, etc.)
- Denture care supplies
- Spare oxygen
- Adult diapers

General health and hygiene:

- First aid kit with over-the-counter medications (see Chapter 4)
- Copies of prescriptions or a printout from the pharmacy
- Face masks for dust or infections
- Shampoo and conditioner
- Deodorant
- Toothpaste and toothbrushes
- Comb and brush
- Lip balm
- Sunscreen and sunglasses
- Spare contact lenses and prescription glasses
- Toilet paper
- Towelettes
- Soap and hand sanitizer
- Liquid detergent
- Feminine supplies
- Plastic garbage bags with ties for personal sanitation use
- Medium-sized plastic bucket with tight lid
- Disinfectant
- Household chlorine bleach

Clothing and bedding:

- Complete change of clothing for each person with extra underwear and socks
- Sturdy shoes or boots; stay away from open toes or heels
- Rain gear, hats, and gloves
- Thermal underwear
- Tent
- Sleeping bag for each person

Safety and communication gear:

- Compass
- Folding shovel
- Waterproof matches or lighter

- Resealable plastic bags of various sizes for all types of non-food uses
- Portable radio or television and plenty of batteries—or an emergency radio that doesn't require batteries (has a wind-up handle)
- Flashlights with extra batteries or wind-up handles
- Whistles for each person
- Fire extinguisher
- Utility knife
- Map with common emergency shelters marked and telephone numbers if available
- Hand-held, two-way radios and extra batteries or chargers

Spare important items:

- Extra house and car keys
- Copies of driver's licenses, work identification, and passports (photocopies are fine)
- Copies of deeds and insurance information
- Copies of vehicle registration and insurance
- Cash and two rolls of quarters for vending machines

Entertainment:

- Games and books to pass the time
- Deck of cards
- Travel games (Scrabble, chess, checkers, Monopoly)
- Crayons and coloring books for the grandkids
- Sudoku/crossword puzzles
- Pens and paper

It's just not possible to pack everything you'll ever need in a kit. We have items we just have to use every day that we can't keep as spares. Make a checklist of what to grab when you go:

- Prescription medications, including inhalers
- Special medical equipment (oxygen tanks, nebulizers)
- Dentures
- Cell phones and chargers
- Driver's licenses or identification cards
- Credit cards
- Favorite dolls or stuffed animals for the grandkids if they are coming along

LIGHTS OUT

For thousands of years of human history we got by just fine without electricity; you'd think we could rough it for a few days without power now. Alas, the reality is we need electricity for our most basic needs. I'm not talking about the TV or the computer here—for me, however, both are basic needs. I'm talking about the very safety of our food and water supply. If you don't have a professionally installed generator available in a disaster, then you need to know how to survive a power failure.

Stuff in the fridge will be fine for a couple of hours without power. After that it gets a little hairy (not the food, the situation).

Fear not a full freezer—it will be safe and everything should stay frozen for 48 hours as long as you don't open the door. If it's not full, however, it takes less time to thaw out. Coffin-style freezers with the lid on top are even better. The more you open the freezer door, the less time food will stay frozen in it.

Food on the refrigerated side has to stay below 40°F (4°C) at all times. If you don't open the door, a typical refrigerator should keep food cold for about 4 hours during a power failure. If the power is expected to be off longer than 4 hours, all eggs, dairy, meat, and fish should be packed into a cooler with ice. Use a quick-read thermometer and throw out any food warmer than 40°F.

Make sure you have an old-fashioned phone in the house with a single cord that plugs into a phone jack. Phone systems and power grids are separate animals, so your phone line might work even when the power is out. Cordless phones have a base station that needs electricity and won't work in a power failure. Cell phones may work; it depends on the cell carrier and whether everyone else is trying to use their cell phones at the same time.

Don't burn anything inside for cooking or heating that's not in a properly installed fireplace or wood stove. Never use an outside grill or barbecue—charcoal or gas—in the house or under a covered porch. Don't run the stove or the oven to stay warm. Any open flame inside the house puts you at risk for carbon monoxide poisoning (and for burning the house down).

The same goes for generators: don't use them in an enclosed space. The best bet for generators is to have them installed professionally before the power ever goes out.

In the summer months, losing power means losing air conditioning (assuming anyone can afford to run the air conditioner anyway). Follow the steps to avoid heat illness in Chapter 24 (read *Don't Get Sick on Hot Days*).

I Think I'll Stay Home for This One

If instead of evacuating you're planning on hunkering down at home for an extended period of time, you want to have enough supplies. Some of the things in an evacuation kit aren't necessary when you're staying home because you don't have to be portable. There's no need for spare walkers or for sleeping bags if you'll be snoozing in your own bedroom.

Plus, since you're not going to be on the move, you can stock up for a whole week instead of just 3 days. Here are the things you'll need if you do not plan to make a run for it:

* Seven gallons of bottled water per person or pet
* Water purification tablets for extra emergency water supplies
* Food for a week that doesn't need water or heat to prepare—don't forget pet food
* First aid kit (Chapter 3)
* Prescription and non-prescription medications
* Manual can opener (or at least battery-operated with spare batteries)
* Flashlight with fresh batteries
* Battery-powered lanterns (avoid candles)
* Battery-powered radio with fresh batteries or one of those wind-up jobs
* Lighter or matches
* Wrenches to shut off water and gas supplies (store them next to the valves)

Disaster Survival at Home

Since you'll be staying in for this disaster and not making a run for it, you'll have to make some adjustments. You won't have unlimited water supplies and you probably won't have emergency services to call upon if you burn the place down or get sick. It becomes very important to watch out for yourself and your loved ones until things get back to normal.

Here are some tips for everyday disaster survival:

* Use disposable cups, plates, and utensils to conserve water
* Don't use candles if you can help it; chemical light sticks and battery-powered lights are the best bet
* Don't use outdoor grills or barbecues indoors; you could give everyone in the house carbon monoxide poisoning

- Use generators only if they're well ventilated to avoid carbon monoxide poisoning (have the generator professionally installed ahead of time for best results)
- Keep a regular phone (one that only plugs into a phone jack and doesn't have a power cord) for use during power failures
- Get a radio and a flashlight or two that don't rely on batteries (the wind-up emergency kind)

WHAT TO DO IF YOU DIDN'T PREPARE

I know how it goes sometimes. You bought this book and the next day a meteor fell from the sky. You didn't have time to get ready—all this advice gone to waste.

Never fear, I've got some tips for you even if you didn't plan ahead. First and foremost: follow orders and get to safety. If you're told to evacuate immediately, don't wait. Get everybody in the car, grab your keys, and go.

If you have some time to pack before evacuating, take identification, cash, prescription medications, blankets or sleeping bags, and any bottled water you have on hand. Take a change of clothes, including spare underwear, socks, long pants, two shirts, sturdy shoes, and take a coat, even in the summer.

If authorities say it's okay to stay in your home, then pack clothes, identification, cash, water, food that doesn't require refrigeration, prescription medications, and sleeping bags to be ready to leave if you must.

Stay informed. Listen to the radio or television for instructions. If you don't have power at home, use a battery-powered radio or your car radio. If you listen to the car radio, don't let the battery run low. Whatever you do, don't run your car in the garage to charge the battery; you will cause carbon monoxide poisoning.

Water will keep you going longer than anything else. Bottled water is best, but there are ways to treat water and make it safe to drink if necessary (see the sidebar, *Water in a Pinch*). Listen to the radio to find out if tap water is safe. To conserve water, use alcohol-based hand sanitizer and disposable utensils, cups, and plates if you have them.

Another way to conserve water is not to drink it. If you have a cupboard full of soda, juice, and sports drinks, drink them. I know we've all been told that caffeinated drinks actually cause us to be more dehydrated, but that's only when the drinks are crazy full of caffeine and you don't drink them very often (see Chapter 24, *How Much Water is Enough?*).

Eat the most perishable food first—the earliest expiration dates. In a power failure, refrain from opening the refrigerator door as much as

WATER IN A PINCH

If you run out of water or you don't have any stored ahead of time, you can use tap water that's trapped in your water heater tank and pipes. Turn off your water inlet (from the municipal supply or the well) and drain what's left in the pipes into a container.

Only use trapped pipe and water heater tank water if your tap water was safe to drink before the disaster started, and only if you haven't run your tap (or flushed your toilet) since officials declared the tap unsafe.

If you run low on water, don't ration it. Drink what you need today and find more tomorrow. Remember that drinking other nonalcoholic beverages counts as water intake, even if they contain caffeine.

Making water safe to drink in your kitchen is not an exact science. There are just too many things that can contaminate the water supply. Be sure to check with officials for guidance if you can. Water purification tablets can be used for most water supplies. They're easier to use than some of the tricks below:

- If you don't have anyone to ask for help, start by examining your water. If it's not clear or there are visible particles, strain the water through paper towels, coffee filters, or—if absolutely nothing else is available—a clean cloth.
- Use one of the following treatments on your tap water (only do this after all your bottled water and other nonalcoholic beverages are clearly going to run out):
  - Boil water in the biggest pot or kettle you can handle. The bigger the pot, the less of your water is lost during boiling. Get it up to a rolling boil for at least 1 full minute. After it cools, pour the water back and forth between two clean containers to aerate it and improve taste.
  - Boiling is your best option, but if heat is not available, chlorinate your water using unscented liquid household chlorine bleach. The bleach should list 5.25% to 6.0% sodium hypochlorite as its only active ingredient. Use 1/8 teaspoon per gallon of water. Put it in a large, clean pot or kettle. Stir and let stand for 30 minutes. If the water does not have a slight bleach odor (ladies are better at detecting odors than men), repeat the chlorination with another 1/8 teaspoon bleach per gallon and let stand another 15 minutes. If it still doesn't smell like chlorine, find another source of water and start over.

possible. If you have ice available, move food from the fridge to an ice chest within 4 hours of losing power. Frozen goods in a full freezer can last as long as 2 days without power—that's a *full freezer*, by the way; stuff will thaw out sooner in a half-full freezer.

Burning Down the House

If you want to stay safe, proper planning is your best bet. What to do in case of a fire is the most overlooked, but easiest planning anyone can do.

Getting out of your house in the case of a fire depends on your physical ability as much as the exits you have available to you. When you were 12 years old, climbing out a second story window was no problem. You probably didn't even need a ladder.

Get Out In a Hurry

Don't stop to get anything

Don't stop to call 911

Don't go back in the house

Today your needs have probably changed, so you should plan in advance how to escape if the smoke alarm goes off.

In this chapter there is a form to help you plan your escape. I recommend you take advantage of it and decide how you'll get out if the smoke alarm starts wailing. To start, make a floor plan of your house:

- Use a fire escape grid (at the end of this chapter)
- Include each floor
- Note all potential exits, including windows
- Designate two ways out for each room
- Draw arrows to show which way to go (like hotels do)
- Designate a meeting spot

My house only has 5 feet from the outside walls to the fence on either side. If flames are poking out both sides of my house, I'm not going to be running through there to get from the backyard to the front. If your house is the same way, designate two meeting places for your family: one in the backyard and one in the front.

Security bars need a quick release handle on the inside. If your house has security bars on the windows to keep bad guys out, make sure they aren't also keeping the good guys in. If you can't open your security bars, they need to be replaced.

LIFE'S little
EMERGENCIES

Fire Escape Planning Grid

Home Address: _____

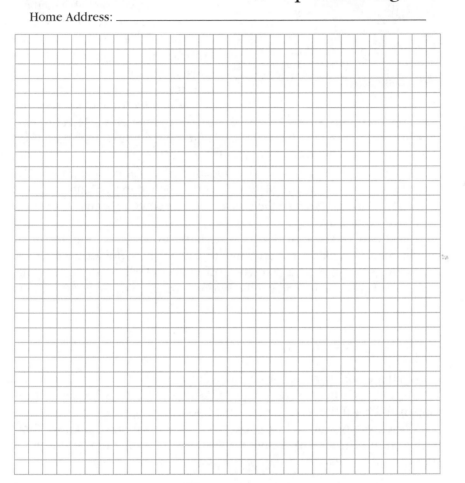

Make a photocopy of this form for each floor of your house. Draw the floor plan on the grid above. Be sure to include all doors and windows. Show the location of all working smoke alarms. Draw arrows to show escape routes. Pick a place for everyone in the house to meet outside.

Practice your escape plan a couple times each year. The best way to make sure you will be safe is to practice getting out of the house *before* a fire happens.

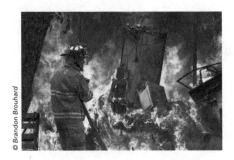

© Brandon Brouhard

Once you have your plan, practice it. There's no such thing as practicing too much. If you have to climb out a window, you probably ought to try at least once before you need to do it for real. You can't hesitate when it's the real thing, so practice with the whole family to make sure you are ready for a fire—or any emergency.

When it is time to go, stay low. Crawling keeps you below the smoke and in the better air. Don't open a door without putting the back of your hand against it first: If it's hot, don't open it. Opening a hot door might let flames rush in.

Once you're out, gather at your meeting place (or places). Take attendance to see that everyone's okay and send someone to a neighbor's house to call 911. *Don't go back in the house,* even if someone is missing. Let the rescuers do that job.

Make sure you have working smoke alarms in every bedroom and in the laundry room. Check the batteries monthly by pushing the little button and change the batteries twice a year when you change clocks for daylight savings time. Also change the batteries if the alarms start chirping every 30 seconds.

FLOODS

Floods affect more parts of the country than any other disaster. If your area is prone to floods, make sure you know how to find out if a flood is going to happen and learn the different levels of flood warnings.

When you're caught in a flood, here's what you need to know about getting around from FEMA and the National Oceanic and Atmospheric Administration (NOAA):

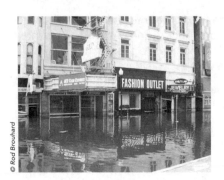

© Rod Brouhard

- If you must walk through water, only go through standing water. Six inches of moving water can sweep your feet out from under you. Use a stick or a cane to check the firmness of the ground in front of you.
- Never drive through a flooded road or bridge. Back up and try a different route.
- Stay on high ground.

Listen to the radio for weather information. Take routes that avoid flooded areas. Information is readily available from the NOAA Weather Radio All Hazards (NWR). Broadcasts require a specific receiver or scanner. It's best to have a receiver with the Specific Area Message Encoder (SAME), which will alert you when flash flood warnings or watches are issued.

There are seven channels (MHz frequencies) used in the NWR:

- 162.400
- 162.425
- 162.450
- 162.475
- 162.500
- 162.525
- 162.550

Do not stay in a flooded car. If your vehicle is surrounded by floodwater, abandon the vehicle and move immediately to higher ground.

If your car is swept into the water and submerged, DON'T PANIC! Stay calm and wait for the vehicle to fill with water. Once the vehicle is full, the doors will open. Hold your breath and swim to the surface.

If you are swept into fast-moving floodwater outside of your car, point your feet downstream. Always go over obstacles, never try to go under.

If you are stranded on something above the floodwater, such as a tree or building, stay put and wait for rescue. Do not enter the floodwater.

Don't overestimate your car's ability to drive through floodwater. Six inches of water is enough to reach the bottom of most passenger cars. Driving in water this deep is enough to cause a loss of control or stall the car. A foot of water will float most cars and 2 feet of rushing water will sweep most vehicles, including SUVs and pickups.

Always avoid contact with floodwater. It can be contaminated with oil, gasoline, or raw sewage. Some of the paramedics and EMTs I worked with after hurricane Katrina got very sick from being in contact with floodwater.

On the Internet

- www.ready.gov
- firstaid.about.com/od/emergencypreparation

29

Traveling Safely

First aid at home is one thing, but traveling safely and knowing what to do if you get hurt on the road is another. In Chapter 2, I talked about using 911 to get help. That advice works as long as you are in the United States. If you go out of the country, however, there's no guarantee that dialing 911 will get you an ambulance. You should always check with the country you are visiting to learn how to summon help if you should get seriously ill or injured.

When traveling on the road, always wear your seat belt. I know many of you reading this book didn't have to wear seat belts when you were learning to drive and some of you never got into the habit at all. Despite the fact that you've lived just fine (so far) without a seat belt, you really should wear one whenever you're in the car.

Although if you don't, I'm not going to complain too loudly. Where I work we call not wearing your seat belt *job security*. Seat belts not only protect you from dying in a car crash, but from sustaining a severe brain injury and other injuries as well. If you don't want to be changed forever, put your seat belt on.

WHERE TO TURN IN AN EMERGENCY ON THE GO

If you're in another country, the medical care you'll get depends on the country you're in. How to get help in another country is also dependent on your location. However, international travel isn't just about being on the ground in another country or even being on dry land at all.

Cruise ships and airplanes are rather popular ways to get around these days. If you find yourself on either of these modes of transportation, potential medical care might depend entirely on who else is on board with you.

Airplanes especially are a challenge. Airplanes do not staff medically trained personnel, beyond the emergency first aid training of the cabin crew (flight attendants). Airplanes do have medical kits with various tools available to help should a medically trained passenger be there to assist you.

I have one recommendation should you find yourself in need of emergency medical care on an airplane (or a train for that matter): instead of a doctor, ask for a paramedic. Paramedics have less training than a doctor, for sure, but our training is very specific to emergency care. Not only that, but we practice our craft in a different place every time we treat a patient. We're used to figuring it out as we go and taking care of folks with serious medical conditions.

If you ask the flight attendant for assistance on board an aircraft, he or she will ask for help over the loudspeaker. You are rolling the dice that someone will be able to help you any time you're trapped on an airplane. In the case of a very serious medical condition, the pilot may decide to land the plane at an alternate airport on the way in order to get you to an ambulance and on to the ER faster. If you can wait, the pilot may decide to proceed to the final destination and just have an ambulance waiting for you there.

911 MIGHT BE SPELLED DIFFERENTLY IN OTHER COUNTRIES

We can thank the United Kingdom for our 911 system. London started the use of a 3-digit, easy-to-remember emergency phone number in 1937. We didn't get 911 up and running until almost 30 years later.

In the United States and Canada, 911 is the number. Here are emergency numbers for the countries Americans travel to most:

- Mexico: 066
- All of Europe: 112 (including the UK, but they still have 999 also)
- Japan: 119 for fire and ambulance, 110 for police
- Hong Kong: 999
- China: 110 for police, 119 for fires, and 120 for ambulances. The number is 999 in Beijing and Shanghai.

Cruise ships are a little different. First of all, you should be spending more time on a cruise ship than you did on the flight there. Because of that, the cruise line will usually have a physician on board who can treat minor illnesses and injuries. In most cases, the function of the cruise ship medical staff is to treat minor injuries or illnesses on board and to stabilize major conditions until the passenger can be moved off the ship. Hardly ever will passengers (or ill crew members) be removed from the ship at sea by helicopter. Instead, patients are transferred off the ship at a port of call—usually wherever the ship was headed in the first place.

All in all, medical care during travel is very much left in your own hands. I recommend talking with your travel agent about options if you're concerned about injury and illness during your trip.

Motion Sickness

Puking should be against the law. I don't know how we would enforce it, but I doubt there are too many feelings worse than nausea. Personally, I'd rather hurt than puke. Interesting fact: the words nausea and nautical come from the same root. Nausea literally means sea *sickness*. Other than making you miserable, I don't understand what function nausea has.

There are plenty of home remedies for nausea, but the best way to fix motion sickness is with medication. Most antinausea medications are antihistamines and many antihistamines (*diphenhydramine* is the most common) can be used in a pinch to calm your tummy. There are several over-the-counter remedies and you can ask a pharmacist for recommendations. The antinausea drug most people seem to prefer is the one that comes in a patch you place behind your ear. That drug, *scopolamine*, is only available by prescription.

On the Internet

- www.sccfd.org/travel.html
- firstaid.about.com/od/travelinjuries

Notes

CHAPTER 2

1. Voice-over Internet Protocol (VoIP) is the type of phone that comes bundled with Internet and television service. If you get your telephone service from a cable company or if your telephone service is bundled together with your television and Internet service, you have VoIP service. If you're not sure, call your phone company and ask them. When buying a medical alert system, it's very important to tell the alarm company if your phone is a VoIP phone. For more information, visit http://www.fcc.gov/voip.
2. http://www.fda.gov/NewsEvents/Newsroom/PressAnnouncements/ucm183247 .htm.

CHAPTER 6

3. In 2004, Lisa Torti pulled her then-friend and coworker Alexandra van Horn from a wrecked car that Torti thought was about to explode. Paralyzed as a result of the accident, van Horn sued both the driver and Torti, claiming, among other things, that Torti's actions caused her injuries. Court rulings from the case resulted in a new Good Samaritan Law for California.

CHAPTER 17

4. Christina Chan and Gohar A. Salam, "Splinter Removal," *American Family Physician* 67, no. 12 (2003): 2557–62.

CHAPTER 21

5. Institute for Clinical Systems Improvement (ICSI), "Adult Low Back Pain," *Bloomington (MN): Institute for Clinical Systems Improvement (ICSI)*; 2008 Nov. 66 p.

6. Dean C. Norman, "Fever in the Elderly," *Clinical Infectious Diseases* 31, no. 1 (2000): 148–51. Epub 2000 Jul 25. Review. PubMed (10913413).

7. A. Atahan Cagatay et al., "The Causes of Acute Fever Requiring Hospitalization in Geriatric Patients: Comparison of Infectious and Noninfectious Etiology," *Journal of Aging Research* 2010 Aug 12;2010:380892. PubMed (21151521); PubMed Central (PMC2989655).

8. Meenu Singh and Rashmi R. Das, "Zinc for the Common Cold," *Cochrane Database of Systematic Reviews*, no. 2 (2011):. Art. No.: CD001364, doi:10.1002/14651858.CD001364.pub3.

9. "West Nile Virus: What You Need To Know." *CDC*. Updated April 18, 2011, accessed April 26, 2011, http://www.cdc.gov/ncidod/dvbid/westnile/wnv_factsheet.htm.

10. "Meningitis." *CDC*. Updated May 12, 2011, accessed April 26, 2011, http://www.cdc.gov/meningitis/index.html.

11. "Shingles." *NIH Senior Health*. Last reviewed: January 3, 2011, accessed April 25, 2011, http://nihseniorhealth.gov/shingles/toc.html (accessed April 25, 2011).

12. "Methicillin-Resistant Staphylococcus Aureus (MRSA) Infections." *CDC*. Last updated April 15, 2011, accessed April 26, 2011, http://www.cdc.gov/mrsa/index.html.

13. R. Vetter, et al. "Skin Lesions in Barracks: Consider Community-Acquired Methicillin-Resistant Staphylococcus Aureus Infection Instead of Spider Bites," *Military Medicine* 171, no. 9 (2006): 830.

14. "CDC Features: Be Food Safe." *CDC*. September 1, 2008, accessed April 26, 2011, http://www.cdc.gov/features/befoodsafe/.

15. Johns Hopkins Medical Institutions. "Norwalk Virus: 'Cruise Ship' Illness Challenging and Costly To Hospitals, Too," *ScienceDaily*, accessed April 26, 2011, http://www.sciencedaily.com/releases/2007/08/070829162751.htm.

16. "The Basics: Clean, Separate, Cook and Chill." *foodsafety.gov*, accessed April 26, 2011, http://www.foodsafety.gov/keep/basics/index.html.

17. Ruth G. Jepson and Jonathan C. Craig, "Cranberries for Preventing Urinary Tract Infections," *Cochrane Database of Systematic Reviews*, no. 1 (2008):. Art. No.: CD001321, doi:10.1002/14651858.CD001321.pub4.

CHAPTER 24

18. Heinz Valtin. "'Drink at Least Eight Glasses of Water a Day.' Really? Is There Scientific Evidence for '8 × 8'?" *American Journal of Physiology. Regulatory, Integrative and Comparative Physiology* 283, no. 5 (2002): R993–1004. Review. PubMed (12376390).

19. Ronald J. Maughan and Jane Griffin, "Caffeine Ingestion and Fluid Balance: A Review," *Journal of Human Nutrition and Dietetics* 16, no. 6 (2003): 411–20. Review. PubMed (19774754).

CHAPTER 26

20. R. Vetter, et al. "Skin Lesions in Barracks: Consider Community-Acquired Methicillin-Resistant Staphylococcus Aureus Infection Instead of Spider Bites," *Military Medicine* 171, no. 9 (2006): 830.
21. Catherine Baxtrom et al., "Common House Spiders Are not Likely Vectors of Community-Acquired Methicillin-Resistant Staphylococcus Aureus Infections," *Journal of Medical Entomology* 43, no. 5 (2006): 962–65.

CHAPTER 27

22. "First Aid Tips." Poison Help. American Association of Poison Control Centers. 2004, accessed March 15, 2007, http://www.1-800-222-1222.info/firstAid/home.asp.
23. J. Routt Reigart and James R. Roberts, *Recognition and Management of Pesticide Poisonings*, 5th ed. (Washington: U.S. Environmental Protection Agency, 1999).
24. "Carbon Monoxide Poisoning: Fact Sheet." *CDC*. Updated April 27, 2009, accessed May 5, 2011, http://www.cdc.gov/co/faqs.htm.

Index